My Thai Chef

Authentic Thai Cuisine for the Western Taste

Trademarks and Rights

Throughout this book, we refer to products and designs which are not our property. These references are meant only to be informational. We do not represent the companies mentioned and were not paid promotional fees. However, if these companies would like to send us evaluation copies of future products, we would be thrilled. References to products are not endorsements, but reflect our opinions in some cases.

COPYRIGHT NOTICE:

My Thai Chef: Authentic Thai Cuisine for the Western Taste

Is published by International Creative Concepts Limited and copyrighted, c 2009 by International Creative Concepts Limited. No part of this book may be reproduced in any form by any electronic or mechanical means (including photocopying, recording, or information storage and retrieval) without permission in writing from the publisher, except for reading and browsing via the World Wide Web. Users are not permitted to mount this file on any network servers.

ISBN: 978-0-578-00942-1

The Authors

Talent Provided by – Chongkonnee Shreebuahchoom, My Thai Chef

Produced and Distributed by – Kevin Thomas, International Creative Concepts Limited

Organization

Thai Appetizers
If it is a meal starter or just a snack, these appetizers are sure to become favorites.

Thai Salads
High in fruits, vegetables and spices we provide a new twist on salad.

Thai Soups
Comfort food or just a warm up for the main course, these soups are an instant classic.

Thai Meals
Noodles, beef, chicken, seafood, we cover it all.

Thai Extras
Desserts, drinks and more. Some special extras to round out your meal.

Contents

INTRODUCTION   1

APPETIZERS   3

SALADS   11

SOUPS   21

MEALS   30

EXTRAS   50

INDEX   55

Introduction

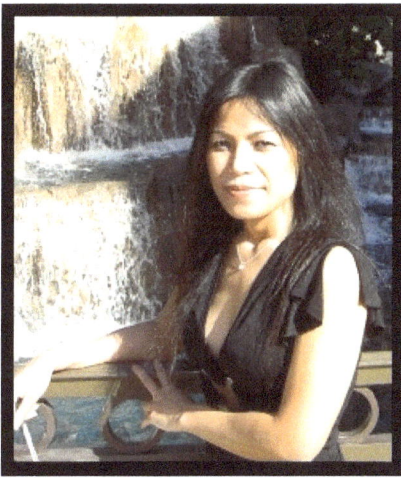

Hello! I am Chongkonnee Shreebuahchoom, founder of My Thai Chef, but everyone can feel free to call me Gee. I was born in Thailand and as a young child I developed the passion for cooking I have today.

As a little one I was not allowed in the kitchen with the older girls and always desired to be like them, telling myself that one day I would have a kitchen of my own.

Since then I have earned a Master's Degrees in business, moved to the United States of America, and now have a kitchen of my own! I have created My Thai Chef so that everyone can bring the joy and tastes of the Thai cuisine to their own home.

Since I have found that many people may find Asian, and more specifically Thai cooking intimidating, I have developed www.mythaichef.com. On this site you will find all of the tools, recipe kits and instructional videos you need to help you prepare any dish in this book.

Often times it is difficult to find the authentic Asian ingredients you need to prepare these recipes. I have also made this easy for you by setting up an online store at www.mythaichef.com where you can come and purchase many of the tools and items you may need.

So please enjoy this cookbook and feel free to email me from www.mythaichef.com if you should have any questions.

Appetizers

This section will address several appetizers that are familiar to the average Thai diet. The specific recipes I have decided to include in this first book are catered towards the western diet.

Not only should many of you should find these recipes easy to prepare but also very appetizing!

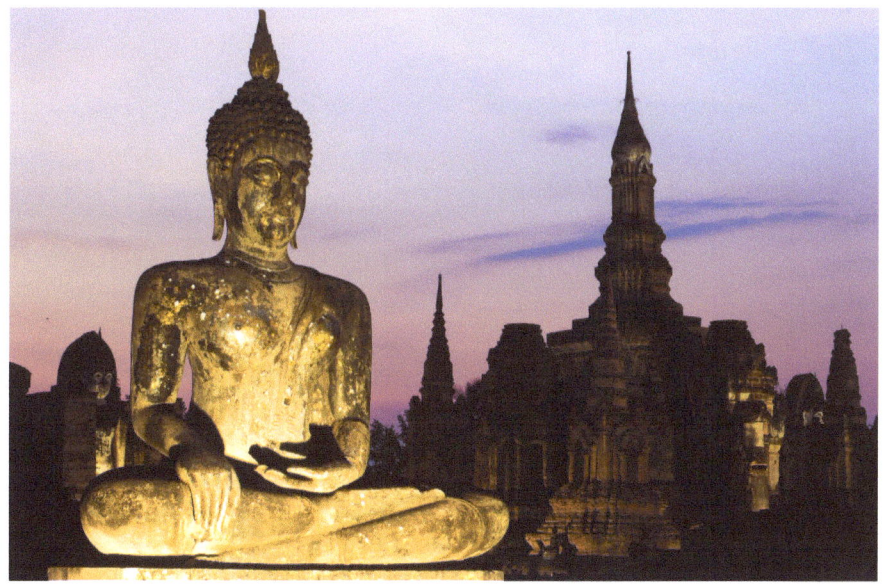

THAI SUMMER ROLLS – are surprisingly easy to make and can be vegetarian, tofu or made with shrimp like in this recipe. Summer rolls are packed with flavor and are a great appetizer for parties.

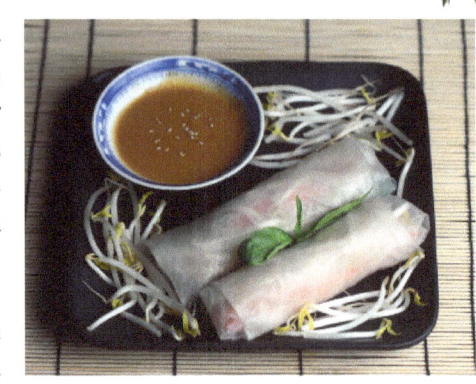

We encourage you to include a dipping sauce of your choice to accompany this dish and have recommended an easy to make Thai dipping sauce.

This recipe will serve 3 – 6 easily   **Prep Time:** 35 Min

Cook Time: 00 Min

6	Medium	–	Spring Roll Wrappers
12	Medium	–	Shrimp, Cooked and Shelled
1	Cup	–	Finely Chopped Lettuce
1/3	Cup	–	Chopped Cilantro
1/2	Cup	–	Cucumber, Peeled, Seeded, Chopped
1	Medium	–	Carrot, Julienned

Note* - Julienning is a method of food preparation in which the food item is cut into long thin strips.

Soak the spring roll wrapper in cool water until limp. Lay the wrapper out flat and place 1/6 of each ingredient down middle of the wrapper, starting with lettuce and ending with the shrimp. Fold over each end and tightly roll the wrapper around the contents, as if making a burrito. Moisten at seam; press to close.

Eat right away or cover with paper towel and refrigerate until ready to serve.

Thai Dipping Sauce – Combine all of the ingredients in a small bowl and serve

1	Tablespoon	–	Light Soy Sauce
1	Tablespoon	–	White-Wine or Rice Vinegar
3	Tablespoons	–	Mirin
1/4	Teaspoon	–	Grated Ginger Root (optional)

Visit www.mythaichef.com/video.html for additional tips!

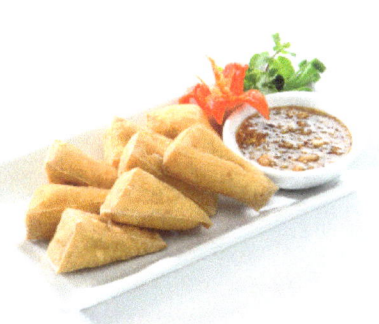

FRIED TOFU – is a vegetarian dish full of protein. Tofu is found throughout the Thai diet and throughout much of Asia.

Tofu can be purchased in soft, medium, firm and extra firm. When preparing the Thai Fried Tofu I recommend you choose a medium to firm Tofu because the soft version will simply fall apart when you go to cook it.

Fried tofu is great on its own or dipped in just about any kind of sauce. My Thai Chef highly recommends a peanut sauce but you may also choose a sweet or spicy chili sauce instead.

This recipe will serve 2 – 4 easily   **Prep Time:** 05 Min

Cook Time: 07 Min

1	block	–	Medium of Firm Tofu
3	Tablespoons	–	Nutritional Yeast
2	Tablespoons	–	Flour
2	Teaspoons	–	Garlic Powder
1/2	Teaspoon	–	Salt
1/2	Teaspoon	–	Pepper
2	Tablespoons	–	Extra Virgin Olive Oil

Slice the block of tofu into even pieces. Feel free to make it easy on yourself and simply cut them into block, but for a better presentation try cutting various shapes such as triangles or circles.

In a bowl combine the yeast, flour, garlic powder, salt and pepper and mix until consistent. Add the tofu to the mixture making sure each piece is coated thoroughly.

In a large pan heat the extra virgin olive oil over medium heat. Once the oil has reached cooking temperature add the tofu. Cook the tofu for 7 minutes or until golden brown and crispy.

Visit www.mythaichef.com/video.html for additional tips!

My Thai Chef

SCALLOPS – are a quick and easy seafood dish that is sure to impress your dinner guests. Thai Scallops are best served on a bed of spinach, lettuce or with fresh Thai herbs.

Also, try adding your favorite hard bread as a nice addition.

Seafood is a staple in the Thai diet as the southern part of the country is boarded on the west by the Andaman Sea and on the south by the Gulf of Thailand.

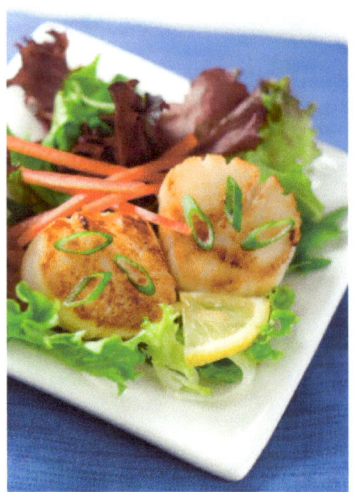

Thai Scallop Sauce

Prep Time: 08 Min

Cook Time: 01 Min

2	Tablespoon	–	High Quality Extra Virgin Olive Oil
1	Tablespoon	–	Tiparos Thai Fish Sauce
1	Tablespoons	–	Freshly Squeezed Lime Juice
1	Large	–	Fresh Red Chili Finely Chopped
1	Clove	–	Fresh Garlic Minced
1/4	Cup	–	Cilantro Finely Chopped

Remove all of the seeds from the fresh large chili before chopping. Once all the ingredients are squeezed, chopped, and minced – mix all of them together in a medium sauce pan and set aside while you prepare the Scallops.

The extra time will allow the garlic and cilantro to soften up in preparation for cooking.

Continue to next page ……….

MY THAI CHEF

<u>This recipe will serve 2 – 3 easily</u>   **Prep Time:** 05 Min

Cook Time: 12 Min

6	Large	–	Sea Scallops
2	Tablespoons	–	Extra Virgin Olive Oil
1	Teaspoon	–	Salt
1	Teaspoon	–	Thai Chili Powder or Black Pepper

Note* - You can choose to season your scallops with hot thai chili powder or the more mild black pepper depending on your taste.

Prepare the Scallops by washing and drying them thoroughly. It is important that the Scallops are very dry in order to achieve the golden brown look in the picture.

Set the heat to medium and add the 2 Tablespoons of extra virgin olive oil to the hot pan allowing the oil to heat up to cooking temperature. You can turn up the heat to medium high to achieve a crispier outside but be careful not to undercook the inside of the scallop.

Place the scallops into the hot oil making sure to space them evenly so they do not touch. Allow the scallops to cook for 4 minutes seasoning the tops of them with a dash of salt and Thai chili powder.

After 4 minutes the first side should be golden brown. Use a spatula or other utensil to gently lift and turn the scallops. Season the scallops once again with the salt and Thai chili powder, and allow to cook for and additional 4 minutes.

Once both sides are golden brown remove the scallops and place them on a paper towel while you cook the sauce you previously set to the side.

Place the sauce onto medium high heat and stir vigorously for only 1 minute. Just long enough to allow the mixture to warm up. After a minuet remove from the heat and add the scallops.

Turn the scallops so that both sides are covered with the sauce mixture. Gently remove the scallops and place them onto the serving dishes you have prepared with your spinach leaves and Thai herbs. – Add a slice of lemon or lime for presentation!

Visit www.mythaichef.com/video.html for additional tips!

SPICY OYSETERS – are identified as a source of virility in the Thai culture. This little dish can be prepared raw or with a quick 1 minute trip in the microwave.

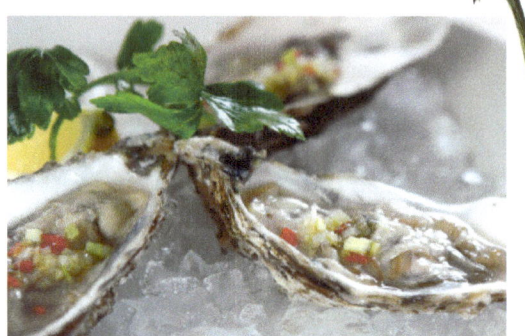

The spicy Thai chili and green onion vinaigrette really brings out the flavor of the oyster.

This recipe will serve 2 – 3 easily   **Prep Time:** 30 Min

                                             Cook Time: 01 Min

1	Dozen	–	Fresh Oysters, With Shell
1/4	Cup	–	Cilantro, Finely Chopped
1	Medium	–	Lemon
2	Tablespoons	–	White Wine Vinegar
1/4	Cup	–	High Quality Extra Virgin Olive Oil
1	Medium	–	Green Onion, Chopped
1	Medium	–	Fresh Red Thai Chili
1	Dash	–	Salt
1	Dash	–	Pepper

Pour the vinegar into a small bowl and whisk in the olive oil in a thin stream. Add Thai chili, green onions, and salt and pepper. Let stand at least 30 minutes to blend flavors.

Clean and shell the oysters discarding only the unused shell. Place the Oysters in a tray of ice to keep cool in preparation for the vinaigrette. Once the vinaigrette has had time to blend poor overtop of the oysters making sure not to overfill. Garnish with the chopped cilantro and lemon juice then serve.

If eating raw oysters does not appeal to you place the oysters in the microwave for 1 minuet before adding the vinaigrette to cook them.

Visit www.mythaichef.com/video.html for additional tips!

My Thai Chef

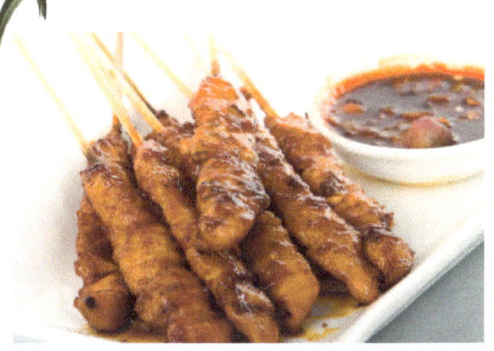

SATAY – is a vey quick and easy appetizer to make for parties or as a quick snack. Satays are typically cooked over the barbeque in many traditional Thai settings, but feel free to use your stove's grill, a flat pan or even the George Forman grill.

The versatility of this dish is only limited by the various sauces you choose to dip it in.

This recipe will serve 2 – 3 easily   **Prep Time:** 30 Min

Cook Time: 10 Min

1	Teaspoon	–	Sugar
1	Teaspoon	–	Salt
1	Pound	–	Lean Pork, Chicken, or Beef
2	Tablespoons	–	Curry Powder
1/2	Cup	–	Coconut Milk
10	Medium	–	Skewers

Note* - There are several curry powder selections you may choose from. For the purposes of this recipe I recommend using *******

To avoid burning the skewers soak them in water for about a half hour before cooking. Do this at about the same time you begin the marinade.

Slice the meat into thin strips that will fit onto the skewers in preparation for soaking. Mix the curry powder, sugar and salt together in a bowl with the coconut milk. Once you have achieved an even consistency add your meat of choice and let soak for approximately 30 minutes.

Thread the meat onto the skewers and let cook for 10 minutes or until thoroughly cooked. Once grilled choose your dipping sauce and serve.

My Thai Chef recommends **peanut sauce** and cucumber in vinegar to accompany this dish. In the Thai Extras section of this book we show you how to prepare a homemade peanut sauce.

Visit www.mythaichef.com/video.html for additional tips!

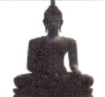 *My Thai Chef*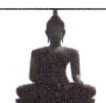

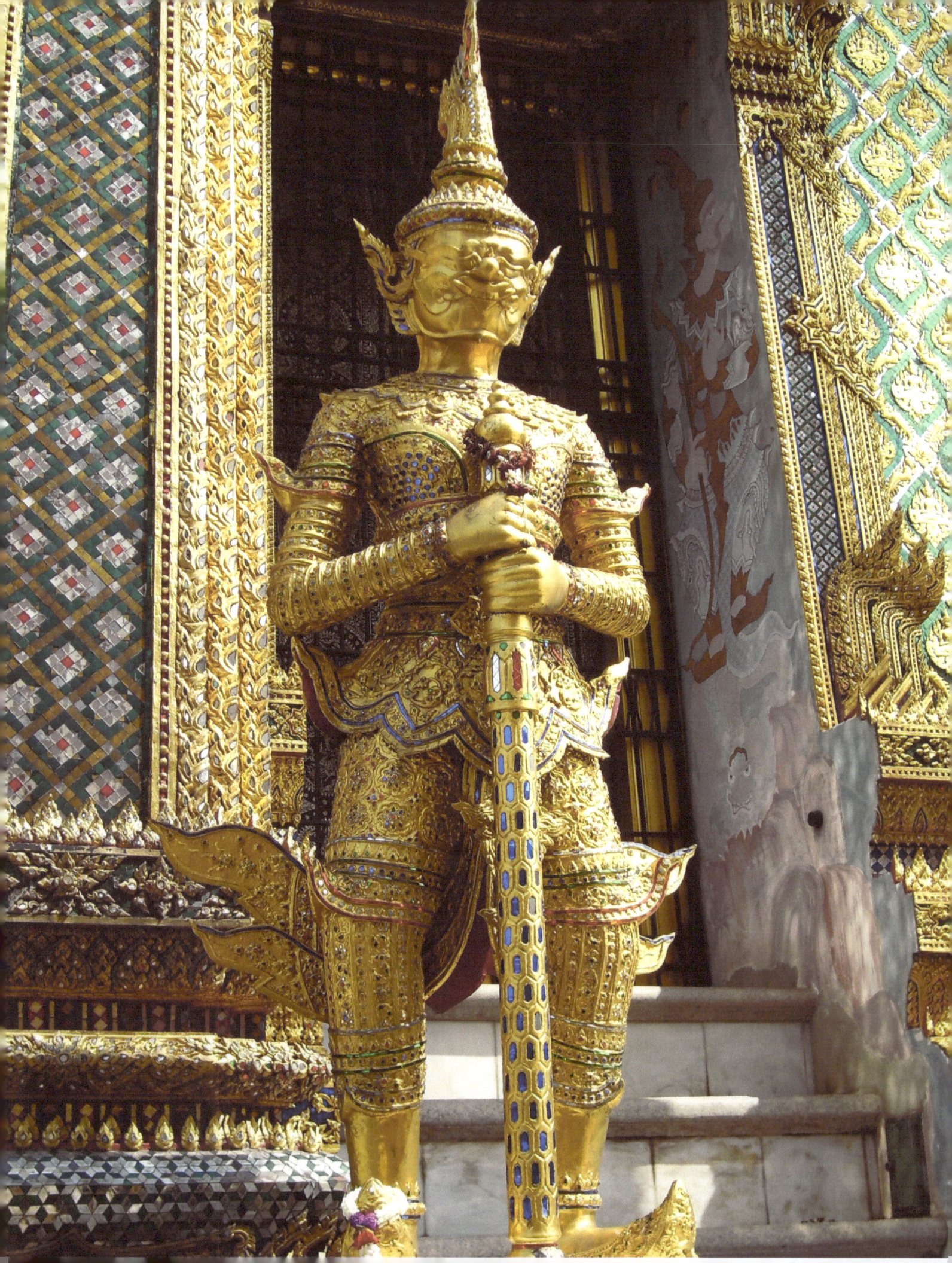

Salads

This section will address several salads that are familiar to the average Thai diet. The specific recipes I have decided to include in this first book are catered towards the western diet. Thai people will often times will exclusively eat salads if they are looking to loose weight.

Not only should many of you should find these recipes easy to prepare but also very appetizing!

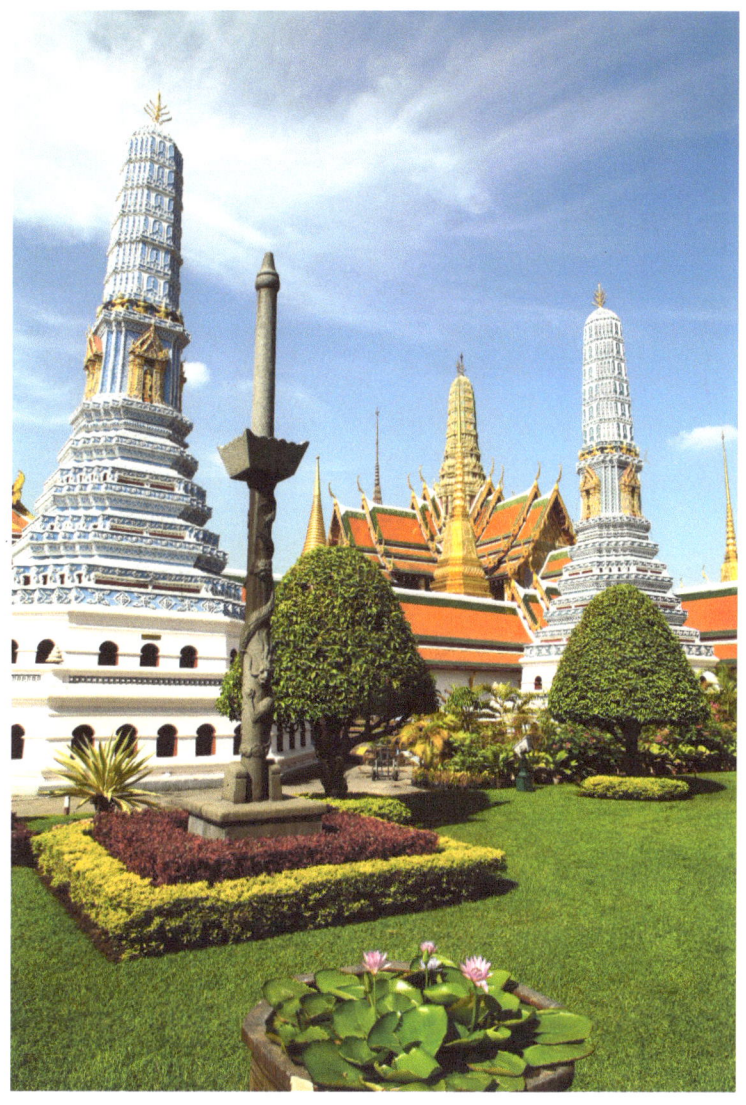

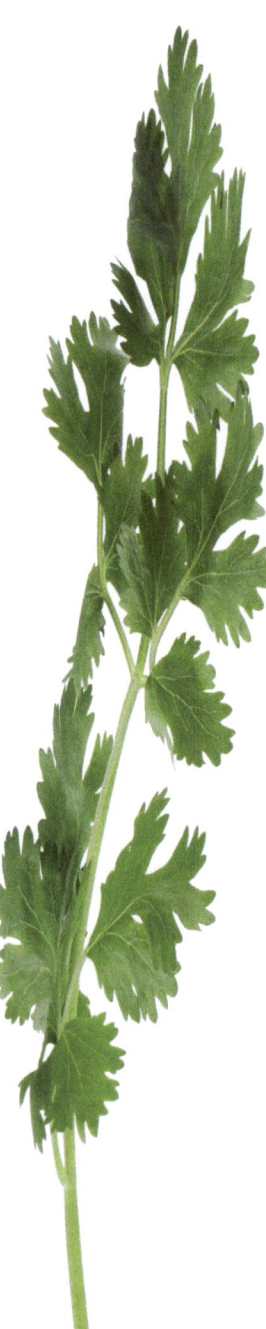

PAPAYA SALAD – is referred to as "Som Tam" in Thai and is famous for being the dish to eat if you want to loose weight.

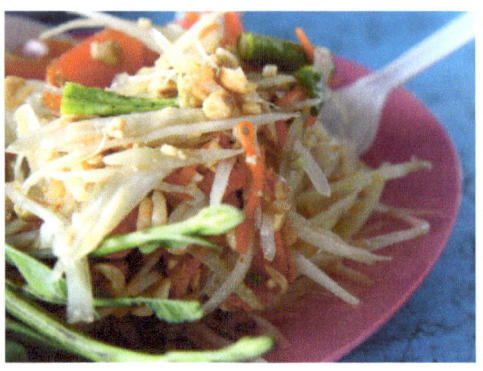

Rich in fresh vegetables this vegetarian salad can be as mild or as spicy as you like.

Papaya salad requires a green unripe papaya which may be difficult to find in your average grocery. Since this is very important My Thai Chef recommends that you go to your local Asian Supermarket to find.

This recipe will serve 2 – 3 easily   **Prep Time:** 30 Min

Cook Time: 00 Min

1 ½	Tablespoons	–	Sugar
1	Medium	–	Lime, squeezed into juice
2	Cups	–	Green Unripe Papaya, Shredded
5	Long	–	Green Beans, Fresh
1	Clove	–	Garlic
1 ½	Tablespoons	–	Tiparos Thai Fish Sauce
2	Medium	–	Thai Chili Peppers
4	Medium	–	Cherry Tomatoes
2	Tablespoons	–	Fresh Peanuts, Toasted

Note* - Traditionally, Thai people like to add dried shrimp to the Papaya Salad recipe. If you would like to add dried shrimp start with 1 to 2 tablespoons to start.

In Thailand papaya salad is prepared in a clay mortar with wooden pestle. This can be found in your local Asian store or it is available for order at mythaichef.com.

Begin by placing the garlic in the mortar and smashing the clove. Once the clove is soft and smashed, begin to add the green beans by cutting them into fourths, followed by the cherry tomatoes which you will cut in half.

Use the wooden pestle to pound the green beans and tomatoes a few times to soften them up. Add the Thai chili peppers and pound them a few times to release the heat into your salad. If you do not like your food spicy omit the Thai chilies all together.

MY THAI CHEF

At this point your mixture should consist of the garlic, green beans, and tomatoes. Now add all of the remaining ingredients. Combine the green papaya, peanuts, lime juice and fish sauce into the mortar and use the pestle and a spoon to mix. Be sure to combine all of the ingredients so the mixture is consistent throughout.

Do not smash the ingredients to the point where they are unrecognizable. The true purpose of smashing is to release the juices and combine the flavors. Once you have all of the ingredients mixed together plate and serve.

Papaya Salad is best served along side roasted chicken or with fried rice.

Keys Items to use for preparation of this meal:

Mortar & Pestle

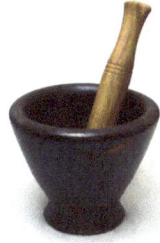

Visit www.mythaichef.com/video.html for additional tips!

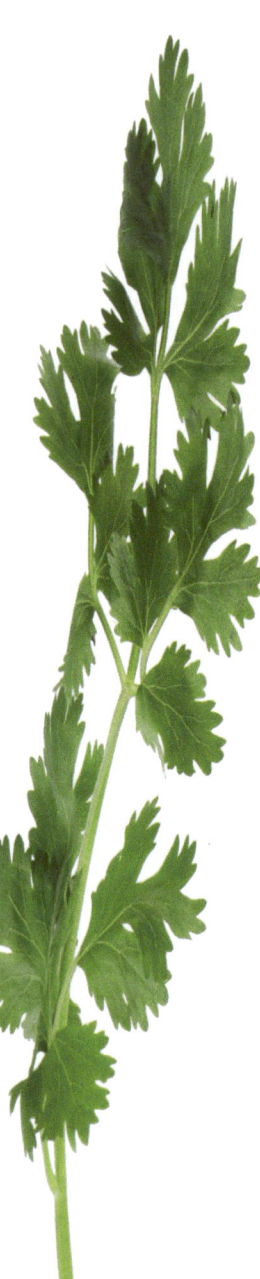

PRAWN SALAD – is referred to as "Pla Goong" in Thai and can also be made with squid or scallops, or any combination of the three.

This salad combines the best of Thai flavors and is another example of the roll seafood plays in the Thai diet.

This is a quick and easy dish that is sure to please even the most sophisticated tastes.

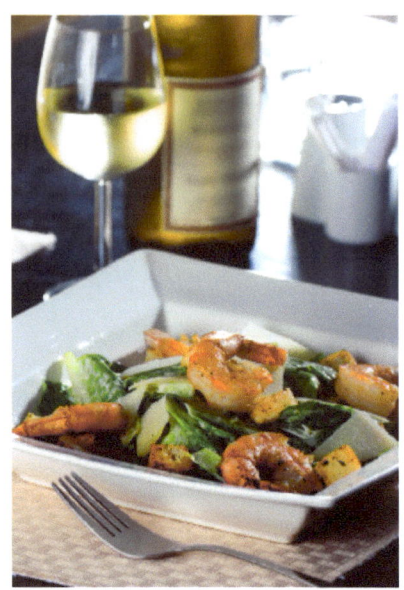

This recipe will serve 2 – 3 easily

Prep Time: 10 Min

Cook Time: 05 Min

1	Pound	–	Prawn Tails
3	Cups	–	Water
2	Tablespoons	–	Lemon Grass, Chopped
1	Tablespoon	–	Lime Leaves, Chopped
1	Tablespoon	–	Cilantro, Chopped
2	Tablespoons	–	Lime Juice
2	Teaspoons	–	Sugar
1	Teaspoon	–	Fresh Garlic, Finely Chopped
1	Teaspoon	–	Ginger Root, Finely Chopped
1/2	Teaspoon	–	Black Pepper
1/2	Cup	–	Green Onions, Sliced
1/2	Cup	–	Mint Leaves

Start by poring the 3 cups of water into a medium sized sauce pan and bring it to a boil.

While you wait for the water to boil prepare the prawn tails by removing the outer shell and cleaning the vein.

Continue to next page ……….

Once the water has come to a boil add the lemon grass, cilantro and lime leaves. Let this mixture boil for 5 minutes.

Once the greens have had time to boil drop in the prawn tails and allow them to cook for only one minute. Be careful not to over cook the prawns, avoiding a rubbery texture.

After 1 minute remove the prawn tails and rinse them off with cold water. This will help to cool the prawn tails quickly and prepare them to be mixed into the dressing.

In a separate bowl combine the lime juice, sugar, ginger, garlic, and black pepper. Continue to mix the ingredients until the sugar is completely dissolved.

Poor the mixture over the prawn tails and toss ensuring they are fully coated.

Now, add the sliced green onions and mint leaves and toss until mixed.

Serve the prawn salad by itself or, as My Thai chef recommends, over a few leaves of lettuce.

Visit www.mythaichef.com/video.html for additional tips!

NOODLE SALAD – is referred to as "Yum Woon Sen" in Thai and is a great cool dish for those hot summer evenings.

Thailand is a tropical region and many of their dishes are served cool to help combat the tremendous heat the get year round.

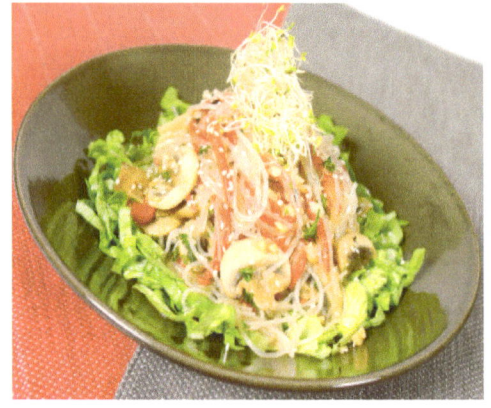

Thai Noodle Salad Dressing

Prep Time: 03 Min
Cook Time: 00 Min

6	Tablespoon	–	Tiparos Thai Fish Sauce
6	Tablespoons	–	Freshly Squeezed Lime Juice
4	Teaspoons	–	Light Brown Sugar
3	Medium	–	Thai Chilies

This recipe will serve 2 – 3 easily

Prep Time: 15 Min
Cook Time: 10 Min

6	Ounces	–	Thai Glass Noodles
1	Pound	–	Ground Chicken
2	Medium	–	Carrots, Julienned
1/2	Cup	–	Celery, Thinly Sliced
2	Small	–	Red Onions, Thinly Sliced
1/2	Cup	–	Green Onions, Chopped
1/2	Cup	–	Cilantro, Chopped
1	Cup	–	Unsalted Peanuts, Roasted
1	Bunch	–	Lettuce, Coarsely Chopped
1	Teaspoon	–	Crushed Red Chili Flakes
1/4	Cup	–	Mushrooms, Sliced

Combine all of the dressing ingredients into a small bowl and taste for the right consistency. Add addition ingredients as needed to suite taste.

My Thai Chef

Once you have mixed to taste set aside for later.

Soak the Thai glass noodles in warm water for about 15 minutes. After the 15 minutes drain the water from the noodles and cut them into smaller lengths. Place the cut noodles into a second bowl and pour hot water over the noodle and soak for an additional 3 to 5 minutes.

Drain the water from the bowl and rinse the noodles in a colander with cold water. Once the noodles are rinsed off let them stand in the colander until ready to add to mixture.

While the noodles are setting in the warm water cook the ground chicken over medium heat adding a bit of water to prevent from burning. Once the chicken has browned removed any excess water and pour the chicken into a large bowl.

Let the chicken cool for about 3 to 5 minutes.

Once the Chicken has cooled add the dressing and toss lightly. Add the cooled noodles and mix completely.

Add the julienned carrot, sliced celery, red onion, green onion, cilantro, mushrooms, and half of the roasted peanuts.

Divide the lettuce onto serving plates and place noodle mixture on top. Sprinkle the remaining roasted peanuts and crushed chili flakes on top of the salads and serve.

Visit www.mythaichef.com/video.html for additional tips!

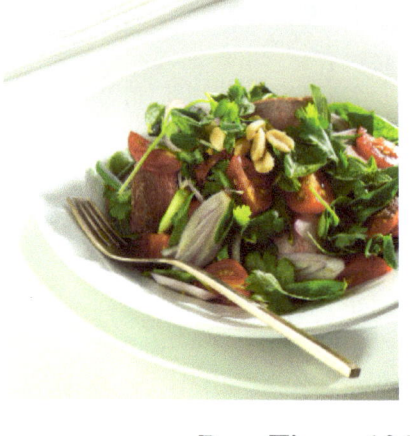

BEEF SALAD – is referred to as "Yum Nua" in Thailand. This spicy little dish can be prepared with grilled or boiled beef.

My Thai Chef recommends that you grill your beef for the best results.

This recipe will serve 2 – 3 easily

Prep Time: 10 Min

Cook Time: 20 Min

16	Ounces	–	Lean Beef
1/2	Cup	–	Sweet Onion
3	Medium	–	Green Onions
2	Tablespoons	–	Lime Juice
2	Tablespoons	–	Tiparos Thai Fish Sauce
1 ½	Teaspoons	–	Sugar
1	Medium	–	Thai Chili, Finely Chopped
1/2	Cup	–	Tomato, Diced or Chopped
1/4	Cup	–	Cilantro, Chopped

There are several ways to prepare the beef but it is important that you grill the beef to achieve the best results. You can do this by broiling the beef on both sides for 2 – 4 minutes or actually grilling the beef. Also, for a quick and easy alternative please feel free to use your George Forman Grill.

Once the beef is cooked, making sure to leave a little bit of red in the middle, thinly slice the beef. Cut the beef at an angle across the grain and in bite size pieces.

Mix the prepared beef with all of the rest of the ingredients in a large bowl. Garnish with the chopped cilantro and serve. Thai Beef Salad is best served along side sticky rice.

Visit www.mythaichef.com/video.html for additional tips!

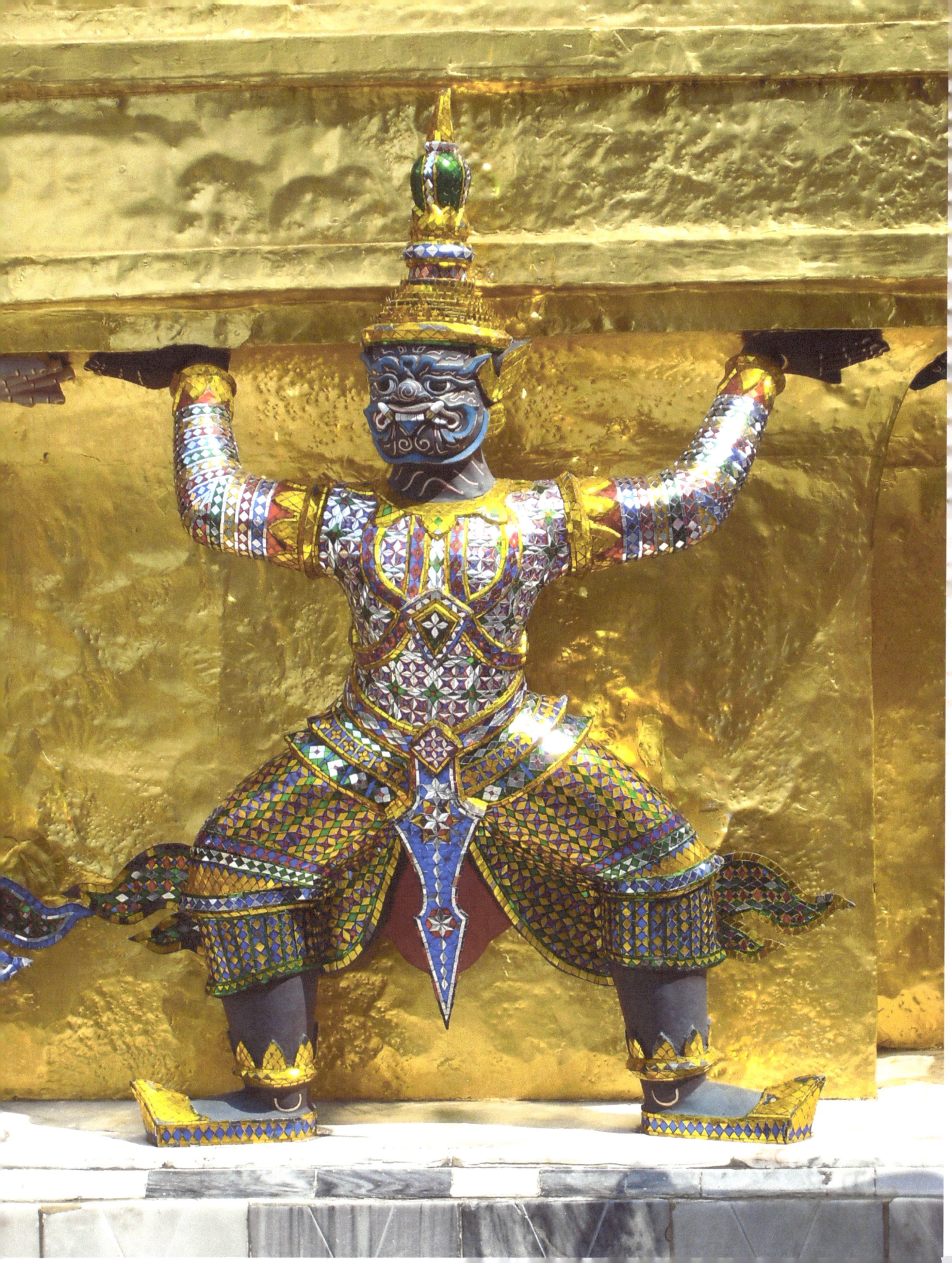

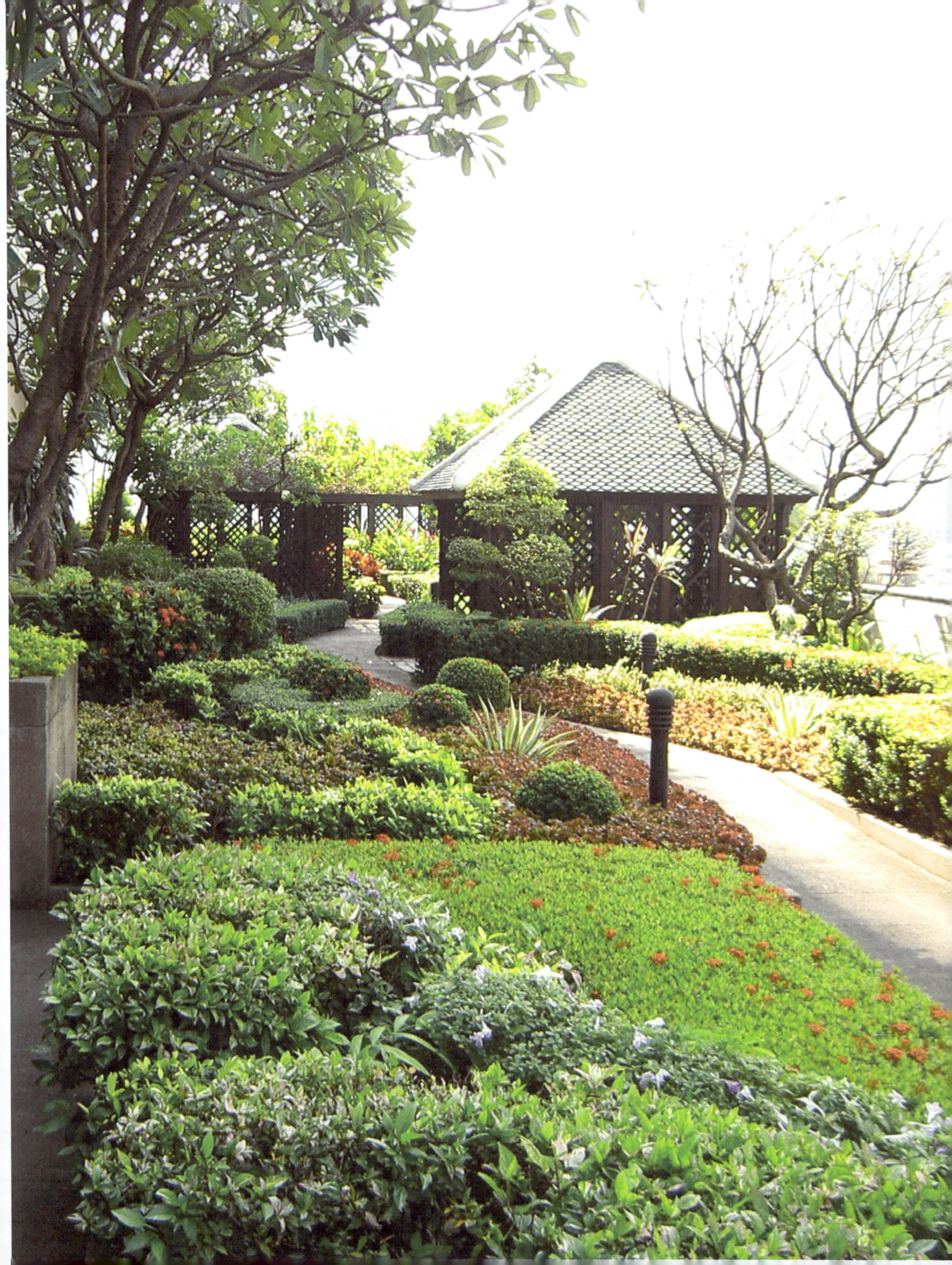

Soups

This section will address several soups that are familiar to the average Thai diet. The specific recipes I have decided to include in this first book are catered towards the western diet.

Not only should many of you should find these recipes easy to prepare but also very appetizing!

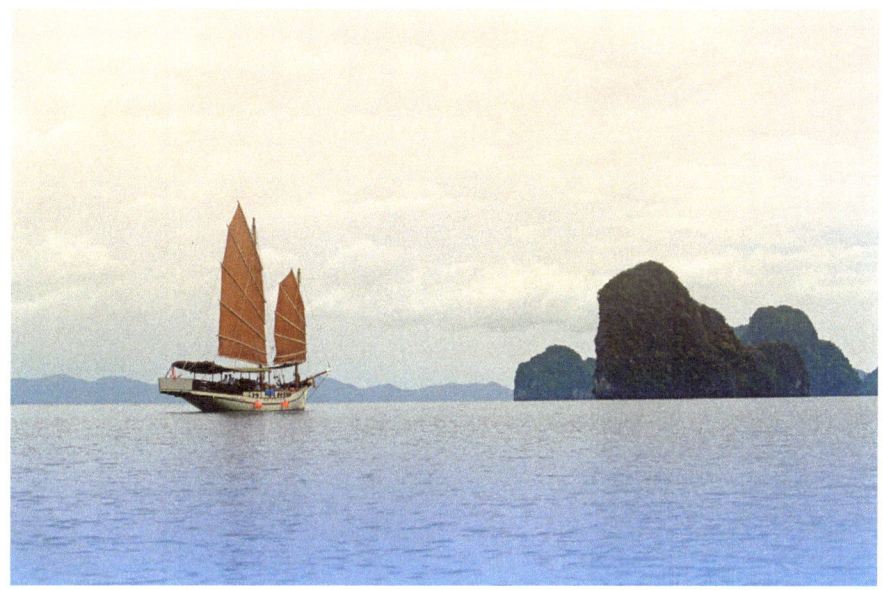

COCONUT CHICKEN SOUP– is referred to as "Tom Kha Gai" in Thai and is a rich, aromatic soup that can be enjoyed as a stand alone meal.

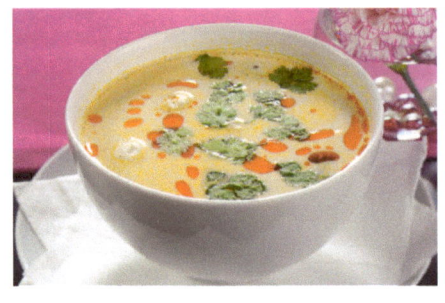

This soup can be prepared with chicken or shrimp.

This recipe will serve 3 – 4 easily

Prep Time: 10 Min

Cook Time: 14 Min

16	Ounces	–	Coconut Milk
6	Thin	–	Galangal, Thinly Sliced
2	Stalks	–	Lemon Grass, Crushed
5	Medium	–	Lime Leaves, Cut in Half
8	Ounces	–	Lean Chicken Breast, Sliced
5	Tablespoons	–	Tiparos Thai Fish Sauce
2	Tablespoons	–	Sugar
1/2	Cup	–	Lime Juice
1	Teaspoons	–	Black Chili Paste
1/4	Cup	–	Cilantro, chopped
5	Medium	–	Green Thai Chili Peppers, Crushed

Start by cutting the lemon grass stalks in to 1 inch lengths using only the bottom third portion of the stalk. Crush the lemon grass with a mortar and pestle to release the aromatic flavors of the lemon grass.

Combine half the coconut milk with the galangal slices, lemon grass and lime leaves in a large saucepan and heat to boiling.

Once the coconut milk mixture has come to a boil add the chicken, fish sauce and sugar. Mix until the sugar is fully dissolved.

Simmer the soup for about 4 minutes, or until the chicken is fully cooked. Add the remaining coconut milk to the saucepan and heat just to boiling.

Place the lime juice and chili paste in a serving bowl then pour the soup into the serving bowl.

Garnish with the chopped cilantro and crushed Thai chili peppers, and serve.

Visit www.mythaichef.com/video.html for additional tips!

My Thai Chef

SPICY CHICKEN SOUP – is referred to as "Tom Yum Gai" in Thai and is a great comfort food. This soup is believed to provide immune boosting benefits and is a very popular hot and spicy soup among Thai people.

This recipe is a great mixture of herbs and spices.

<u>This recipe will serve 3 – 4 easily</u>   **Prep Time:** 15 Min

Cook Time: 15 Min

1	Pound	–	Lean Chicken Breast, Cut into Pieces
3	Cups	–	Chicken Stock
3 1/2	Ounces	–	Canned, Straw Mushrooms
6	Medium	–	Cherry Tomatoes, Cut in Half
1	Medium	–	Lemon Grass, Cut into Short Lengths
2	Medium	–	Lime Leaves, Chopped
3	Tablespoons	–	Tiparos Thai Fish Sauce
4	Tablespoons	–	Lime Juice, Freshly Squeezed
1/2	Teaspoons	–	Sugar
5	Medium	–	Red Thai Chili Peppers, Crushed

Pour the chicken stock into a medium sauce pan and add the lemon grass and lime leaves and heat to a boil. Turn the burner to medium heat to ensure the bottom does not burn.

Add the chicken breast pieces, mushrooms, fish sauce, lime juice and sugar to the soup. Cook for about 10 minutes without stirring the soup.

After 10 minutes of cooking add the tomatoes and red chilies and cook for an additional 5 minutes.

Feel free to garnish with chopped cilantro or sliced green onions for added flavor.

Visit www.mythaichef.com/video.html for additional tips!

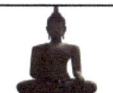 *MY THAI CHEF*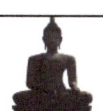

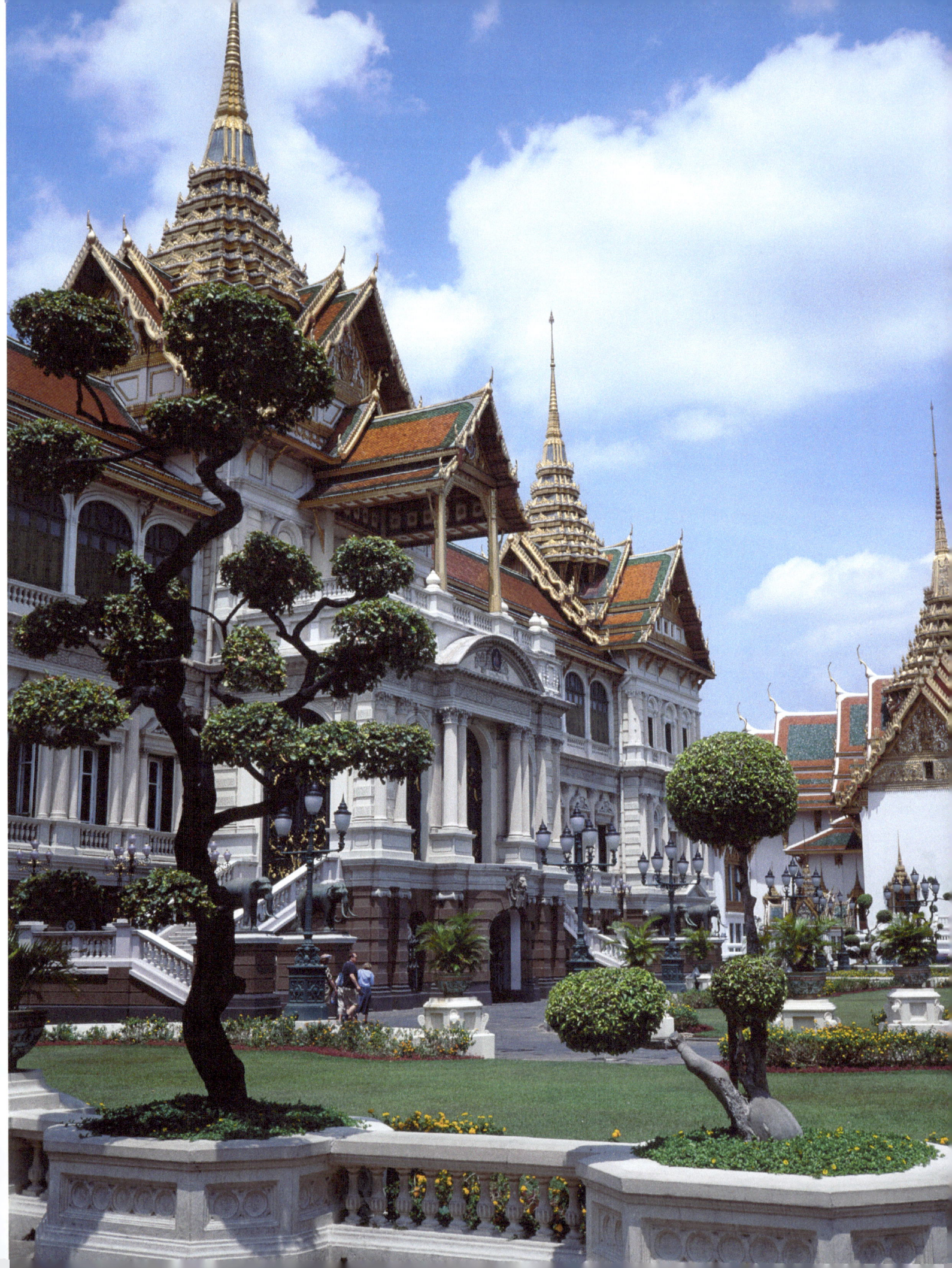

SPICY SHRIMP SOUP – is referred to as "Tom Yum Taleh" in Thai and is a seafood soup very popular in southern Thailand.

This quick and easy dish takes less than 30 minutes to prepare and is right in herbs and spices.

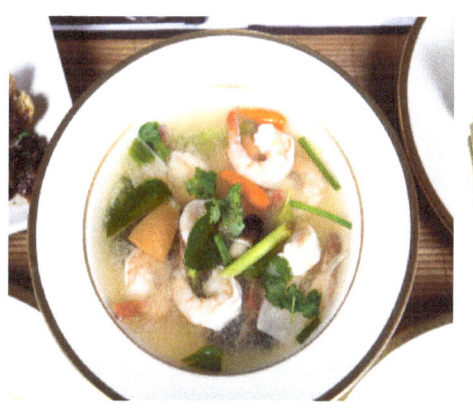

This recipe will serve 3 – 4 easily

Prep Time: 15 Min
Cook Time: 15 Min

1/4	Pound	–	Medium Sized Shrimp
3	Cups	–	Water
3	Cloves	–	Garlic, Smashed
6	Medium	–	Cherry Tomatoes, Cut in Half
1	Medium	–	Lemon Grass, Cut into Short Lengths
3	Medium	–	Lime Leaves, Chopped
2	Tablespoons	–	Tiparos Thai Fish Sauce
4	Tablespoons	–	Lime Juice, Freshly Squeezed
2	Teaspoons	–	Sea Salt
5	Medium	–	Red Thai Chili Peppers, Crushed

Bring the water to a boil add the lemon grass, sea salt, and garlic letting boil for 4 minutes. There should be enough water to cover the shrimp and other ingredients once added.

Add the shrimp, lime juice, chopped lime leaves, and Thai chilies and boil for an additional 2 minutes. Add the fish sauce slowly and taste to seasoned preference.

Add the tomatoes and remove from heat.

You can feel free to make this dish more authentic by adding mackerel and/or squid to the ingredients. Fresh shrimp are the best if you are lucky enough to have access to them.

Visit www.mythaichef.com/video.html for additional tips!

My Thai Chef

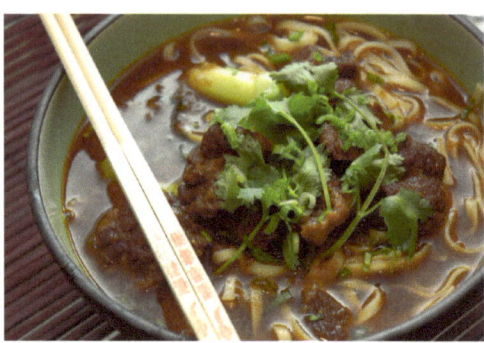

BEEF NOODLE SOUP - is referred to as "Keuteauw" in Thailand and is a real comfort food. The mixture of fresh vegetables, rice noodles, and beef make this more of a meal than a soup.

This recipe will serve 3 – 4 easily

Prep Time: 15 Min
Cook Time: 45 Min

1/4	Pound	–	Beef Bone, Soup Bone
1/2	Pound	–	Beef, Thinly Sliced
1	Package	–	Thai Rice Noodles, Thin
3	Medium	–	Garlic Cloves
1	Teaspoon	–	Salt
2	Tablespoons	–	Sugar
2	Tablespoons	–	Tiparos Thai Fish Sauce
3	Tablespoons	–	Beef Paste
1	Teaspoons	–	Black Pepper Corn, Smashed
4	Medium	–	Green Onions, Chopped
1	Bunch	–	Cilantro, Chopped
1/2	Pound	–	Bean Sprouts
1	Medium	–	Celery Stalk, Chopped

Boil water in the big pot and add beef bone, salt, smashed garlic, sugar, fish sauce, smashed whole black peppercorn and beef paste. Boil on medium heat for about 30 minutes.

Soak dry noodles about 10 minutes in cold water and drain then cover with plastic wrap. Once the soup base has boiled for 30 to 45 minutes then boil water in a separate pan. Place the noodles in the pan for 2 minutes or until lightly soft. Strain and put into serving bowl.

Now add the beef slices to your ladle and put into boiling base for a few minutes until cooked. Remove from soup base and add to serving bowl.

Now that you have the noodles and beef in the serving bowl add a tea spoon of vinegar, handful of cilantro, green onions and bean sprouts.

Now, to finish the dish pour the boiling soup base over all the ingredients in your serving bowl. Ladle just enough soup base to cover the noodles and to see the vegetables float.

You can add some of crushed red Thai chili pepper if you want to spice up your dish, adding more fish sauce or sugar for a saltier or sweeter taste.

Visit www.mythaichef.com/video.html for additional tips!

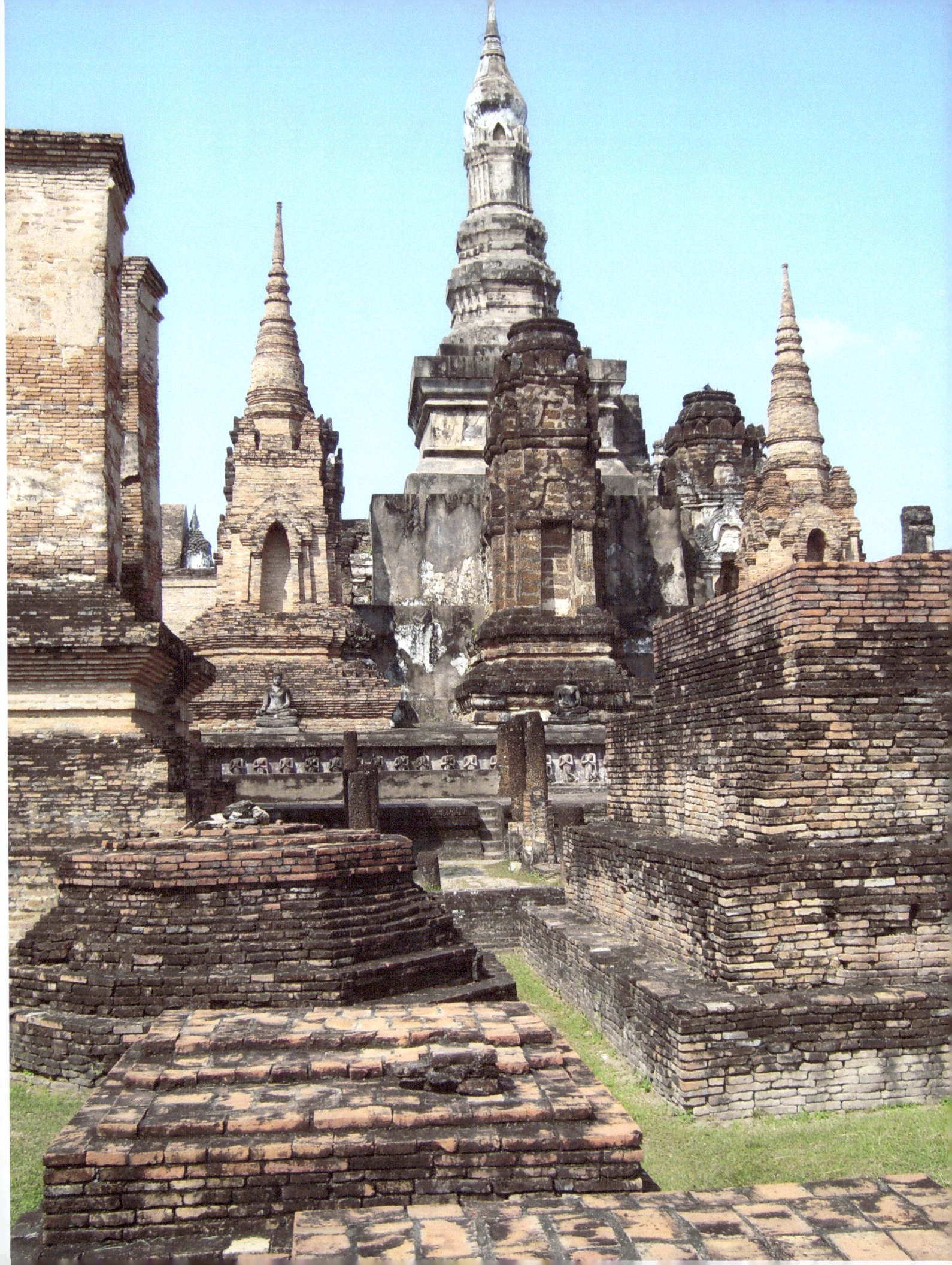

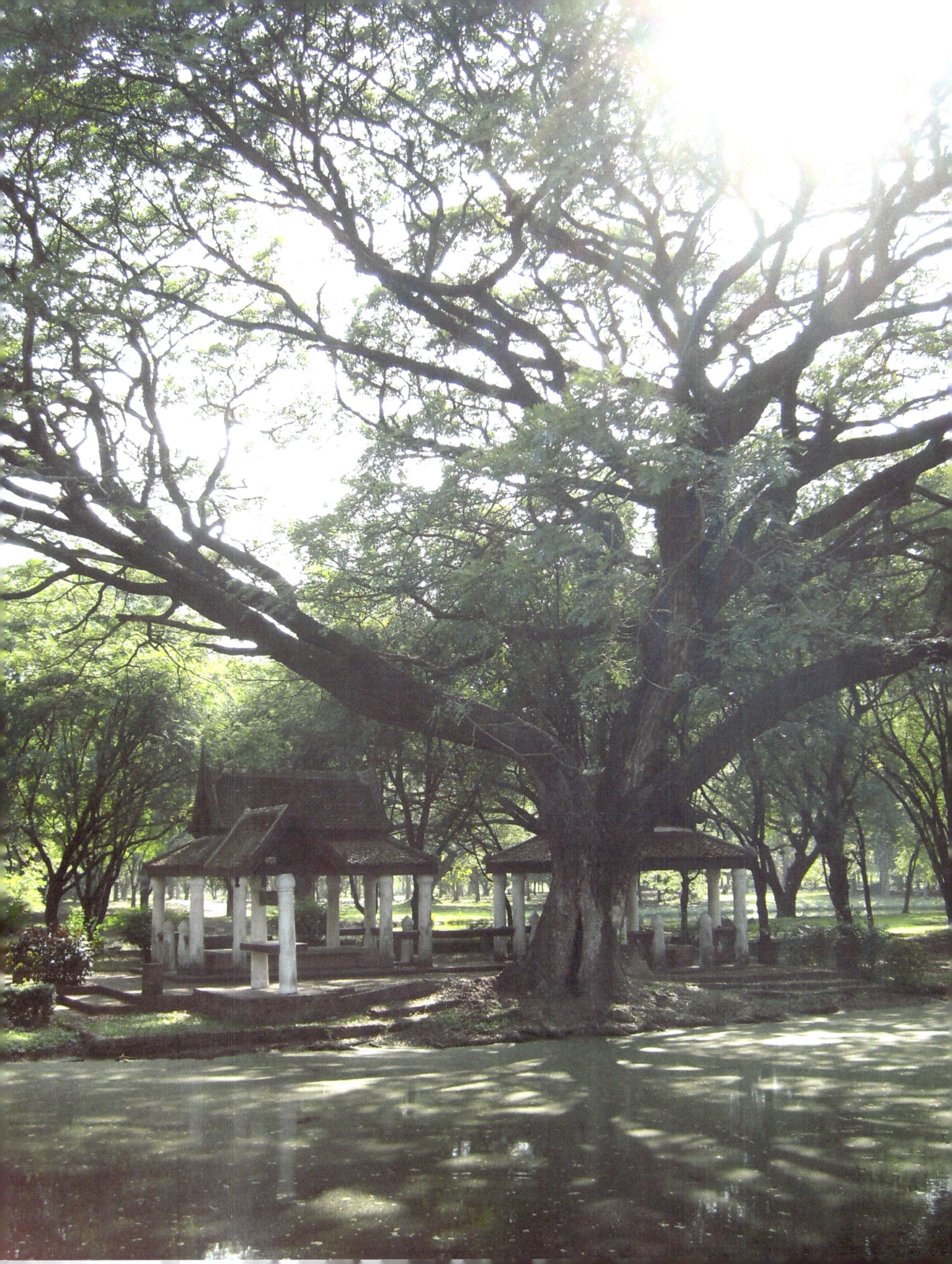

Meals

This section will address several meals that are familiar to the average Thai diet. The specific recipes I have decided to include in this first book are catered towards the western diet.

Not only should many of you should find these recipes easy to prepare but also very appetizing!

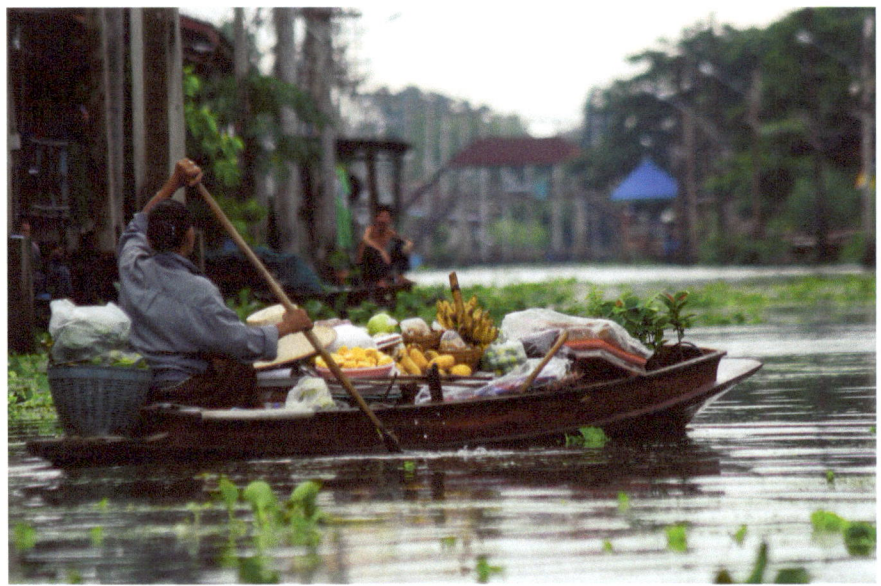

THAI SPICY FISH – is referred to as "Pla Rad Prik" in Thai and is a crispy fried fish topped with a good mix of flavors.

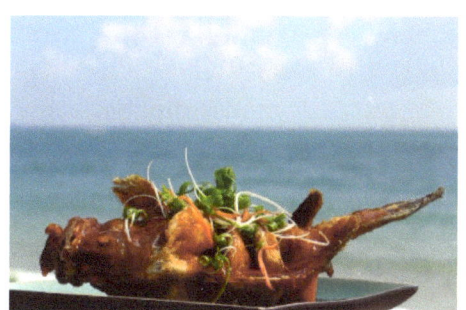

This is a "can't loose" recipe with the sauce My Thai Chef has included.

Thai Spicy Fish Sauce

Prep Time: 03 Min
Cook Time: 00 Min

3	Tablespoon	–	Garlic, Finely Chopped
1/4	Cup	–	Green Thai Chili, Thinly Sliced
1/4	Cup	–	Red Thai Chili, Thinly Sliced
1/4	Cup	–	Red Thai Chili, Thinly Sliced
1/4	Cup	–	Green Onion, Chopped
1/4	Cup	–	Cilantro, Chopped
1	Tablespoon	–	Sugar
1/4	Cup	–	Basil Leaves, chopped
1	Sprinkle	–	Freshly Ground Peppercorn

This recipe will serve 1 – 2 easily

Prep Time: 15 Min
Cook Time: 10 Min

1	Pound	–	Fresh Tilapia or Red Snapper Whole
1/4	Cup	–	Rice Wine or White Wine
1	Cup	–	Plain Flour
1	Quart	–	Canola Oil for Frying

Begin by preparing the sauce in a medium sized sauce pan. Add some oil to the hot sauce pan and stir fry the chilies and onions until soft. Add the fish sauce and bring to a slight boil.

Continue to next page ……….

Once the mixture has come to a slight boil add the sugar and stir until completely dissolved. Add the cilantro leaves and still occasionally until slightly reduced. This should take about 5 minutes.

Remove from the heat and transfer to a serving dish.

Once cooled add the basil leaves and peppercorn.

Pour the oil into a deep pan or deep fryer and heat to 250 degrees. This would be medium high on the stove.

Prepare the fish for cooking by removing all of the insides and scaled. Many fish markets will do this for you in advance of purchase.

Now, cut three for four slashes in both sides of the cleaned fish.

Sprinkle the fish with rice wine and dust liberally with flour, ensuring the fish is fully covered.

Place the fish into the hot oil and deep fry until crispy on both sides.

Remove the fish from the oil and allow to dry on a paper towel doing your best to remove any excess oil. Place the fish on a serving dish and pour the sauce you prepared earlier over top of the fish.

Garnish the fish with cilantro, green onions and bean sprouts and serve.

Visit www.mythaichef.com/video.html for additional tips!

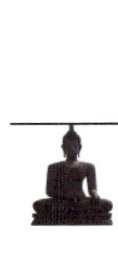

MY THAI CHEF

SEAFOOD CURRY – is referred to as "Ho Mok Talay" in Thai and is a dish with tremendous flavor. For those of you who love seafood and curry this dish is the one for you.

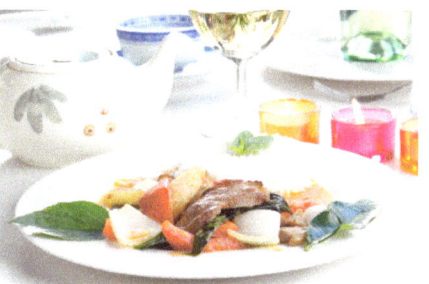

This dish is best severed along side a helping of rice.

Thai Curry Paste   **Prep Time:** 03 Min
                                         Cook Time: 01 Min

2	Medium	–	Lemon Grass, Cut into Short Lengths
2	Thin	–	Galangal, Thinly Sliced
2	Medium	–	Red Onions, Thinly Sliced
1	Clove	–	Garlic, Crushed or Minced
2	Teaspoons	–	Shrimp Paste
1	Teaspoon	–	Lime Peel, Shredded
5	Medium	–	Red Thai Chili Peppers, Dried

This recipe will serve 2 – 3 easily   **Prep Time:** 15 Min
                                         Cook Time: 10 Min

1	Cup	–	Cleaned and Cooked Shrimp
1	Cup	–	Cooked Red Snapper
1	Large	–	Egg, Beaten
1/2	Cup	–	Coconut Cream
1	Cup	–	Soft Coconut Meat, Thinly Sliced
2	Tablespoons	–	Milk
1/2	Cup	–	Sweet Basil
2	Tablespoons	–	Tiparos Thai Fish Sauce
1/2	Teaspoon	–	Sugar

Continue to next page ……….

My Thai Chef

To begin combine all of the ingredients in the Thai Curry Paste and ground them together. For the best results use a mortar and pestle as your tool for grinding the paste together.

Once the paste is completed heat a pan over medium heat and add olive oil. Once the oil is heated to temperature cook the curry past for about 30 seconds.

After 30 seconds add the coconut cream and stir.

Once the consistency is even, add the prepared shrimp and snapper meat. Add the fish sauce and sugar to taste, adding more or less to your preference.

Finally, add the coconut meat and beaten egg to the mix. Stir for consistency then add the milk and sweet basil.

Cook the final mix for a few more minutes and then serve.

Seafood curry is best served along side a dish of rice or flat bread.

Visit www.mythaichef.com/video.html for additional tips!

MATSAMAN CURRY – is a dish that is often found in the southern part of Thailand. This dish employs a host of dry spices and has a heavy Indian influence.

The curry past can be purchased but My Thai Chef recommends preparing a fresh curry paste on your own and has provided the directions to do so.

However, if you wish to purchase the paste and cannot find it locally you can purchase it from the store on www.mythaichef.com

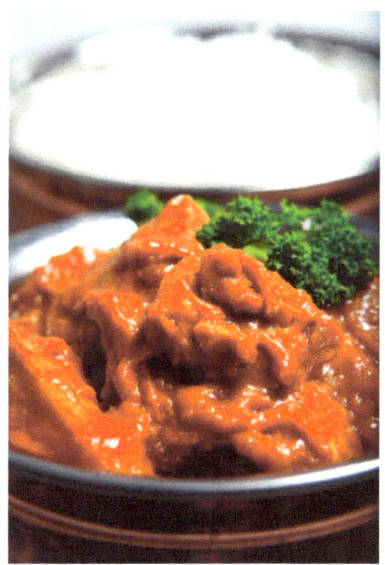

Thai Massaman Curry Paste

Prep Time: 05 Min
Cook Time: 10 Min

10	Medium	–	Red Thai Chili Peppers, Dried
1/2	Teaspoon	–	Peppercorns, Roasted
1	Teaspoon	–	Cilantro or Coriander Seeds, Roasted
1	Teaspoon	–	Cumin Seed, Roasted
2	Medium	–	Cloves, Roasted
2	Medium	–	Cardamom Pods, Roasted
1	Teaspoon	–	Shrimp Paste
1/2	Teaspoon	–	Powdered Nutmeg
1	Teaspoon	–	Salt
1	Teaspoon	–	Magroot Skin
1	Teaspoon	–	Galangal, Minced
1	Tablespoon	–	Cilantro of Coriander Roots, Minced
1	Tablespoon	–	Lemon Grass
1/4	Cup	–	Shallots
2	Tablespoons	–	Garlic, Minced

Continue to next page ……….

My Thai Chef is very impressed if you have decided to make your own paste. To begin start by roasting all of the dry spices over medium heat. It is best to roast each one separately but if you need to save time you can roast them together.

It should take 2-4 minutes to bring out the aroma from the dry spices letting you know when it is done.

Next brown the dry chilies on each side and roast the shrimp paste. To roast the shrimp past you simply wrap the past in tin foil and cook over medium heat.

Once you have roasted the dry chilies soak them briefly in warm water. Separate out the seeds and chop them as finely as you can.

Now you are ready to begin making the curry paste. Start by grinding all of the dry spices you roasted with your mortar and pestle. If you do not have a mortar and pestle at home, you can get one at your local Asian store or from the shop on www.mythaichef.com.

Once the dry spices are ground put to the side for later.

Now put the red chilies into the mortar and pestle and grind until there is a uniform consistency. Continue to pound the chilies adding in all of the remaining ingredients starting with the hardest and working your way to the softest. Do not add the shrimp paste at this time.

Once you have added all of the ingredients and the paste shows even consistency add in the dry spices you set to the side earlier.

Finally, add the shrimp paste to the mix and continue mixing until there is a uniform consistency throughout.

Continue to next page ……….

The ingredients below will be used for the bulk of the Matsaman Curry dish.

<u>This recipe will serve 2 – 3 easily</u>　　　**Prep Time:** 15 Min

Cook Time: 30 Min

4	Tablespoons	–	Prepared or Bought Curry Paste
3	Tablespoons	–	Vegetable Oil
1	Pound	–	Lean Chicken Breast, Cubed
1	Cup	–	Coconut Cream
1	Cup	–	Coconut Milk
1	Cup	–	White Potatoes, Cubed
1	Cup	–	Onions, Coarsely Chopped
4	Medium	–	Cardamom Pods
1/4	Cup	–	Peanuts, Roasted
1	Tablespoon	–	Sugar
1	Inch	–	Cinnamon Stick
2	Medium	–	Cassia or Bay Leaves, Dried
2	Tablespoons	–	Tiparos Thai Fish Sauce
2	Tablespoons	–	Tamarind Paste

Start by cutting the potatoes and onions into smaller pieces. Cubed potatoes are best for consistent cook times (1 in by 1 in cubes).

Wash the chicken clean and cut into bite sized pieces. If you are interested in a more authentic taste substitute the chicken breast for chicken legs and thighs.

Add the hot oil to a pan cooking on medium high. Add the prepared or purchased curry past and fry for 3 to 4 minutes. Continually stir the paste to ensure that it does not burn.

Now, add the chicken pieces to the pan and cook for about 2 to 3 minutes. Here we want to be sure to sear the chicken on both sides.

Once the chicken is seared add the coconut cream to the pan and cook for an additional 2 to 3 minutes. You will want the oil to separate from the coconut and begin to see the reddish paste float to the top. If you cannot find coconut cream you can simply skim the thick cream from a can of coconut milk.

Continue to next page ……….

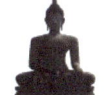 *My Thai Chef*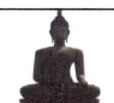

Once the coconut cream has thinned out you can add the potatoes, peanuts and onions to the pan, along with the 1 cup of coconut milk. Allow this mixture to cook on medium low heat for a few minutes.

Finally, add the cinnamon, cardamom seeds, and cassia leaves to the mix and simmer for 15 to 20 minutes.

If the dish begins to get too dry add a little bit of water. When you get close to the end of the cook time, the last 2 minutes or so, add the remaining ingredients. The fish sauce, sugar and tamarind juice are used to add flavor to the dish. Add each of these to taste adjusting for your preference.

When finished serve over rice for the best results.

Many of the dry ingredients for this recipe can be purchased from the store on www.mythaichef.com if you are having a difficult time finding them locally.

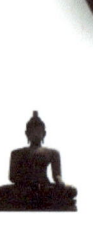

Visit www.mythaichef.com/video.html for additional tips!

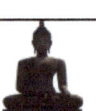

PINEAPPLE SHRIMP CURRY – referred to as "Gang Kua Sapparod Goong" in Thai is a sweet and sour dish that really highlights the imagination of the Thai cuisine. This recipe uses shrimp as its meat base but you can feel free to try mussels or fish.

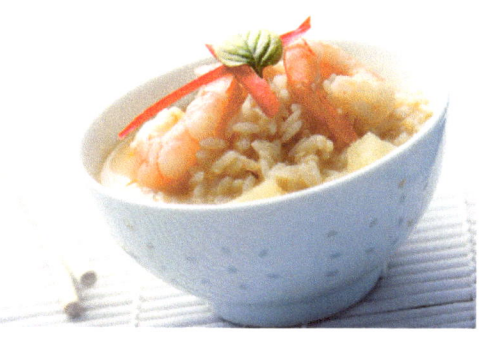

This recipe will serve 3 – 4 easily

Prep Time: 10 Min
Cook Time: 15 Min

2	Cup	–	Coconut Milk
1	Cup	–	Fresh Pineapple, Crushed
2	Tablespoons	–	Red Curry Paste
1/4	Cup	–	Tiparos Thai Fish Sauce
2	Tablespoons	–	Sugar
12	Medium	–	Shrimp, Cleaned and Deveined

Combine all of the ingredients except the shrimp into a large saucepan. Bring the mixture to a boil over medium heat.

Now, add the shrimp to the mixture and allow the curry to come to a second boil. Cook the shrimp for about 3 minutes making sure not to overcook.

Remove from heat and serve. Pineapple Shrimp Curry is best served with rice and My Thai Chef recommends jasmine rice over plain white rice.

Visit www.mythaichef.com/video.html for additional tips!

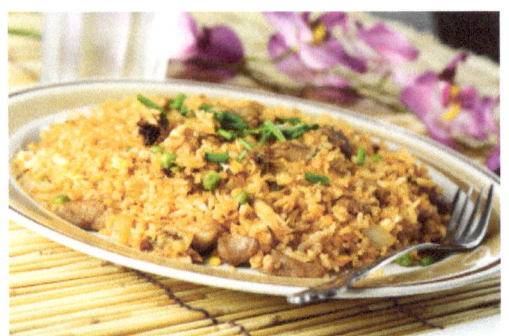

CHICKEN FRIED RICE
– is a great dish that is well known throughout Asia. The Thai version of this classic dish is sure to become one of your favorites.

This recipe will serve 3 – 4 easily

Prep Time: 10 Min

Cook Time: 15 Min

2	Cup	–	Jasmine Rice
1/4	Cup	–	Vegetable Oil
1	Medium	–	Sweet Onion, Chopped
2	Cloves	–	Garlic, Crushed
1	Small	–	Red Thai Chili, Chopped
1/2	Pound	–	Chicken Breast, Chopped & Cooked
2	Medium	–	Eggs, Beaten
1	Tablespoon	–	Cilantro, Chopped
3	Small	–	Green Shallots, Chopped

Fried rice in the Thai tradition is best prepared with rice that is a day old. Prepare the 2 cups of Jasmine Rice and set in the refrigerator over night. You can skip the 1 day wait if you are in a hurry to prepare this delicious meal but be sure to thoroughly drain the cooked rice.

Heat a pan over medium-high heat and add the vegetable oil to the pan. Once the oil has been heated to temperature add the onions and cook until soft. Follow this same step next adding the garlic and chili pepper.

Now, add the cooked chicken (shrimp or pork) and rice to the pan and cook mixing all of the ingredients together. Cook for 3 to 5 minutes or until the rice is thoroughly heated.

Finally, add in the eggs making sure to stir quickly so the egg cooks fully. Remove from the heat and top off with the cilantro and chopped shallots.

Visit www.mythaichef.com/video.html for additional tips!

MY THAI CHEF

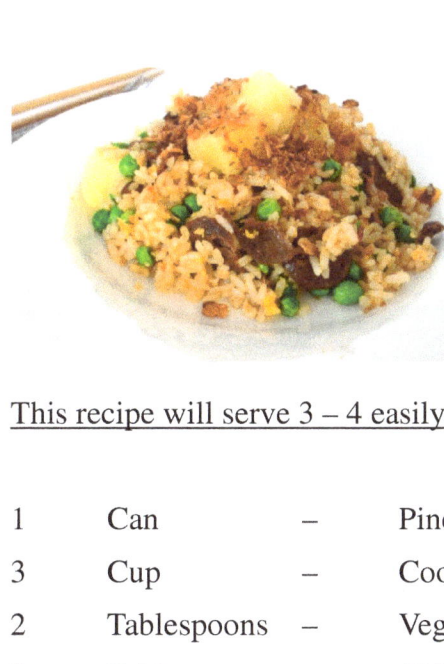

PINEAPPLE FRIED RICE
– is a very popular vegetarian dish in Thailand. In southern Thailand pineapple is as popular a crop as corn is in the United States. This sweet fruit finds its way into many traditional Thai dishes.

This recipe will serve 3 – 4 easily

Prep Time: 30 Min
Cook Time: 10 Min

1	Can	–	Pineapple Chunks
3	Cup	–	Cooked Rice, 1 Day Old
2	Tablespoons	–	Vegetable Oil
2	Tablespoons	–	Chicken Stock
2	Small	–	Shallots, Thinly Sliced
3	Cloves	–	Garlic, Minced
1	Medium	–	Red Thai Chili
1	Medium	–	Egg
1/2	Cup	–	Peas
1/4	Cup	–	Carrot, Grated
1/2	Cup	–	Peanuts, Roasted and Unsalted
3	Medium	–	Green Onions, Finely Chopped
1/3	Cup	–	Cilantro, Chopped
2	Tablespoons	–	Tiparos Thai Fish Sauce
2	Teaspoons	–	Curry Powder

Prepare the rice by adding 1 tablespoon of the vegetable oil and mixing until all the clumps are removed. Set to the side and heat 1 tablespoon of vegetable oil in a pan on medium high heat.

Once the oil has heated to temperature add the shallots, garlic, and Thai chili, and cook for about 1 minute. Keep the pan from drying out by adding chicken stock when needed.

Crack the egg and cook quickly moving it around in the pan. When the egg is cooked add the carrot, peas, and peanuts and cook for an additional minute.

My Thai Chef

Mix the fish sauce and curry powder in a separate bowl and then add to the stir fry mix. Now add the rice and pineapple and cook for additional 3 minutes. You want to cook the rice until it turns golden in color and begins to pop in the pan.

After 3 minutes remove from the heat and serve. Garnish the plated fried rice with the cilantro and green onions.

Visit www.mythaichef.com/video.html for additional tips!

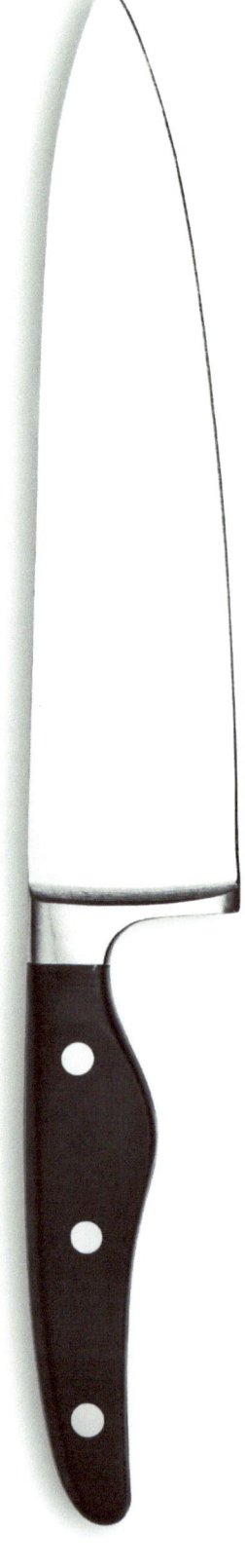

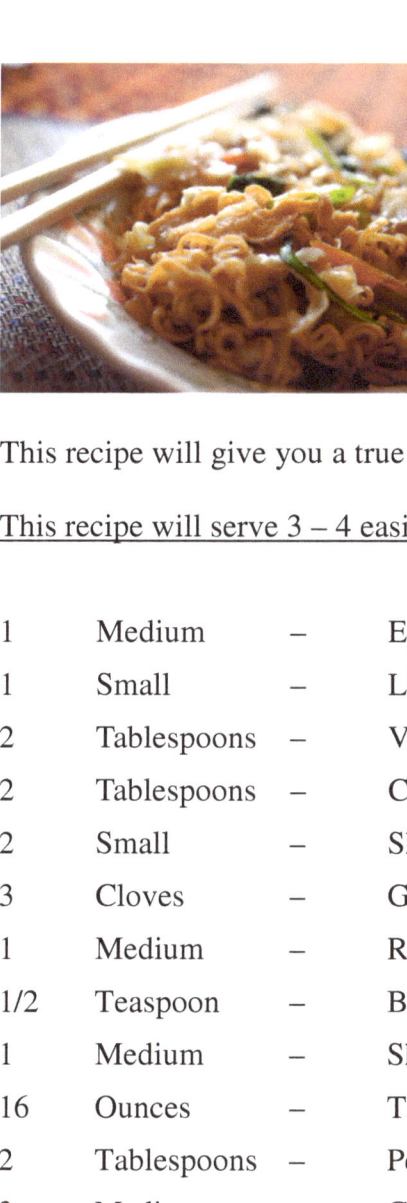

CHICKEN PAD THAI – is a staple dish in the country of Thailand. On almost every street corner you can find Pad Thai and nowhere will you find the red colored Pad Thai you see in many western restaurants.

This recipe will give you a true authentic take on this great dish.

<u>This recipe will serve 3 – 4 easily</u>

Prep Time: 30 Min
Cook Time: 10 Min

1	Medium	–	Egg
1	Small	–	Lime, Juiced
2	Tablespoons	–	Vegetable Oil
2	Tablespoons	–	Chicken Stock
2	Small	–	Shallots, Thinly Sliced
3	Cloves	–	Garlic, Diced
1	Medium	–	Red Thai Chili, Dried & Ground
1/2	Teaspoon	–	Black Pepper
1	Medium	–	Shallot, Minced
16	Ounces	–	Thai Rice Noodles, Wide Cut
2	Tablespoons	–	Peanuts, Roasted & Crushed
3	Medium	–	Green Onions, Finely Chopped
1/3	Cup	–	Cilantro, Chopped
4	Tablespoons	–	Tiparos Thai Fish Sauce
2	Tablespoons	–	Sugar
2	Tablespoons	–	Tamarind
2	Tablespoons	–	Vegetable Oil
1/2	Pound	–	Chicken, Cubed and Cooked
1/3	Cup	–	Extra Firm Tofu, Cubed
1	Cup	–	Bean Sprouts

Continue to next page ……….

My Thai Chef

Begin by soaking the Thai rice noodles in warm water for about 10 minutes. Do this first so the noodle will be ready when it comes time to add them to the pan for cooking.

Cook the cubed chicken fully and set to the side. (You can also substitute the chicken for shrimp)

Prepare the green onions, garlic, and shallot by chopping them and setting them to the side. Save half of the green onions for later to garnish the dish.

Prepare the Tofu by cutting the larger block into several miniature blocks. About ½ inch by ½ inch.

Heat a pan over medium-high heat and add the vegetable oil. Once the oil has reached cooking temperature add the tofu, garlic and shallot and cook until all sides of the tofu are golden brown.

Now its time for the noodles, make sure they are fully drained and add them to the pain keeping the existing ingredients. To keep the mix from burning stir quickly. Add tamarind, sugar, fish sauce, and chili pepper.

If the noodles have added too much moisture you will need to turn up the heat. Pad Thai is a dry dish so do your best to cook out any loose fluids.

You are now ready to add the egg. The trick to cooking the egg is to push all the noodles to one side of the pan. This should leave about half of the pan to cook the egg. Pour the egg into the second half of the pan and scramble until cooked. Once the egg is cooked begin mixing it into the rest of the noodles.

Finally, add the chicken you cooked earlier, half of the green onions, half of the bean sprouts and mix a few more times.

Now plate the Pad Thai and garnish with green onions, bean sprouts, and peanuts.

Visit www.mythaichef.com/video.html for additional tips!

PAN FRIED NOODLES

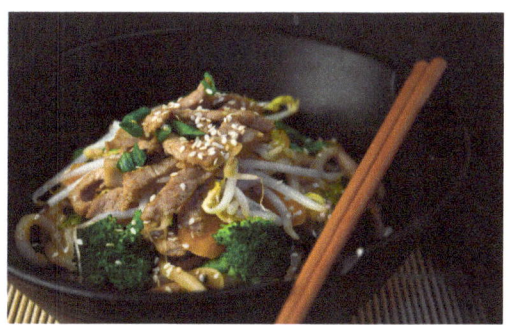

– is referred to as "Pad See-Yew" in Thai and is a versatile dish that can be prepared with chicken, pork or beef.

For this recipe we will be using lean cuts of pork.

This recipe will serve 3 – 4 easily

Prep Time: 10 Min

Cook Time: 15 Min

2	Tablespoons	–	Tiparos Thai Fish Sauce
1	Tablespoon	–	Miso Bean Paste
1	Tablespoon	–	Oyster Sauce
1	Tablespoon	–	Sugar
1/4	Cup	–	Soy Sauce
1	Pound	–	Broccoli, Cut to Pieces
12	Ounces	–	Thai Rice Noodles, Dry Wide Cut
1/4	Cup	–	Vegetable Oil
3	Tablespoons	–	Vegetable Oil, Second Serving
12	Ounces	–	Lean Pork, Thinly Cut
3	Cloves	–	Garlic, Diced
2	Medium	–	Eggs, Beaten
3	Medium	–	Red Thai Chili, Thinly Sliced
2	Tablespoons	–	Peanuts, Roasted & Crushed

Begin by mixing the fish sauce, miso, oyster sauce, sugar and soy in to a large bowl.

Steam the broccoli for about 2 minutes until slightly tender.

In a medium pot boil water and add the Thai rice noodles. Allow the noodles to cook for only 5 minutes as you want them to remain somewhat firm.

Continue to next page ……….

My Thai Chef

cDrain the noodles and rinse under cold water. Be sure to fully dry the noodles before adding to the frying pan.

Transfer the noodles to a large bowl and toss with 1 tablespoons of vegetable oil.

Heat 1 tablespoon of the vegetable oil in a large skillet. Add the pork, season with salt and cook over medium high heat until fully cooked. This should take 2 to 3 minutes to prepare.

Now, remove the pork from the pan and set aside for later. Add the ¼ cup of vegetable oil and heat to cooking temperature.

Add the garlic and cook for about 30 seconds.

Add the beaten egg to the cooked garlic and scramble for another 30 seconds.

Add the noodles to the eggs and garlic and toss lightly.

Add the fish sauce, miso, oyster sauce, sugar and soy mixture to the pan and toss lightly.

Cook this mixture for about 5 minutes doing your best to evaporate all of the remaining liquids.

Continue to cook the noodles for an additional 2 minutes, stirring them until they are golden brown.

Add the broccoli and cooked pork and cook until fully heated.

Remove from heat and serve, garnishing with the peanuts and Thai chilies. You may also add sesame seeds to the top for extra presentation.

Visit www.mythaichef.com/video.html for additional tips!

MY THAI CHEF

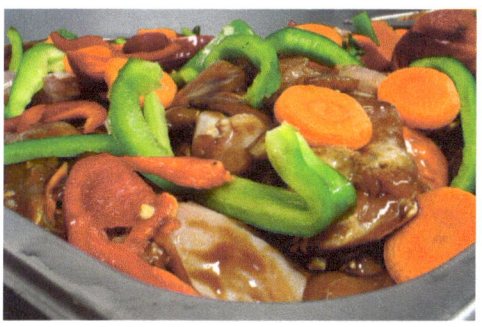

BEEF STIR FRY - is referred to as "Pad Gra Praw" in Thai and mixes fresh vegetables and beef cooked as a stir fry with oyster sauce.

The reference to Ga Praw highlights the Thai basil that is so prevalent in many Thai stir fry recipes.

This recipe will serve 3 – 4 easily   **Prep Time:** 10 Min

Cook Time: 15 Min

2	Cloves	–	Garlic, Sliced
1/4	Cup	–	Tiparos Thai Fish Sauce
3	Tablespoons	–	Thai Basil Leaves
1	Tablespoon	–	Oyster Sauce
1	Tablespoon	–	Curry Powder
3	Medium	–	Red Thai Chili, Thinly Sliced
2	Tablespoons	–	Sugar
1	Pound	–	Beef, Thinly Sliced
1/2	Medium	–	Red Bell Pepper
1/2	Medium	–	Green Bell Pepper
2	Tablespoons	–	Shallots, Thinly Sliced
1	Medium	–	Carrot, Thinly Sliced

Begin by grinding the garlic, shallots, and curry powder into a paste with your mortar and pestle.

Prepare the carrot, bell pepper, Thai chili, and shallots and set them to the side.

Put the paste into a medium sized skillet, & stir-fry the paste over medium heat until thick.

Add in the beef & the remaining ingredients & stir fry until the beef is fully cooked. Remove from heat and serve with a side of rice.

Visit www.mythaichef.com/video.html for additional tips!

MY THAI CHEF

SWEET AND SOUR CHICKEN – is referred to as "Whan Preaw Gai" in Thai and combines the sweet taste of pineapple to stir fry.

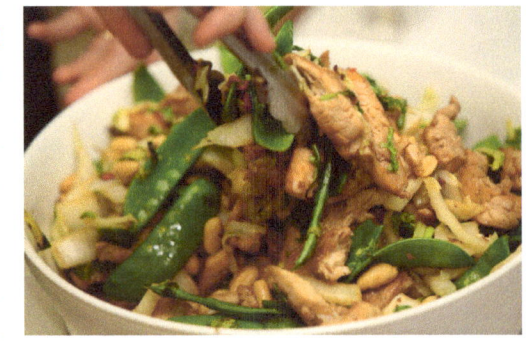

In Thailand pineapple is as popular a crop as corn is in the United States. This sweet fruit finds its way into many traditional Thai dishes.

This recipe will serve 3 – 4 easily

Prep Time: 10 Min

Cook Time: 15 Min

9	Tablespoons	–	Ketchup
3	Tablespoons	–	Vinegar
4	Tablespoons	–	Sugar
1	Tablespoon	–	Vegetable Oil
2	Cloves	–	Garlic, Crushed
1	Pound	–	Chicken Breast, Cut into Chunks
1	Small	–	Onion, Thinly Sliced
2	Medium	–	Red Bell Pepper, Cut into Chunks
12	Ounces	–	Freshly Chopped Pineapple, or 1 Can
6	Ounces	–	Snap Peas, Sliced
1/4	Cup	–	Cashews, Lightly Roasted

Begin by mixing the ketchup, vinegar, sugar and garlic into a small bowl. Mix thoroughly and set to the side for later.

Heat a skillet over medium- high heat and add the vegetable oil. Once the vegetable oil is hot add the chicken, onion and bell peppers to the pan and cook until the chicken is fully cooked.

Now, stir in the mixture you set aside earlier, adding the pineapple and snap peas to the skillet. Cook for an additional 5 minutes.

Remove from the heat for a few minutes before adding the cashews and serve along side rice.

Visit www.mythaichef.com/video.html for additional tips!

My Thai Chef

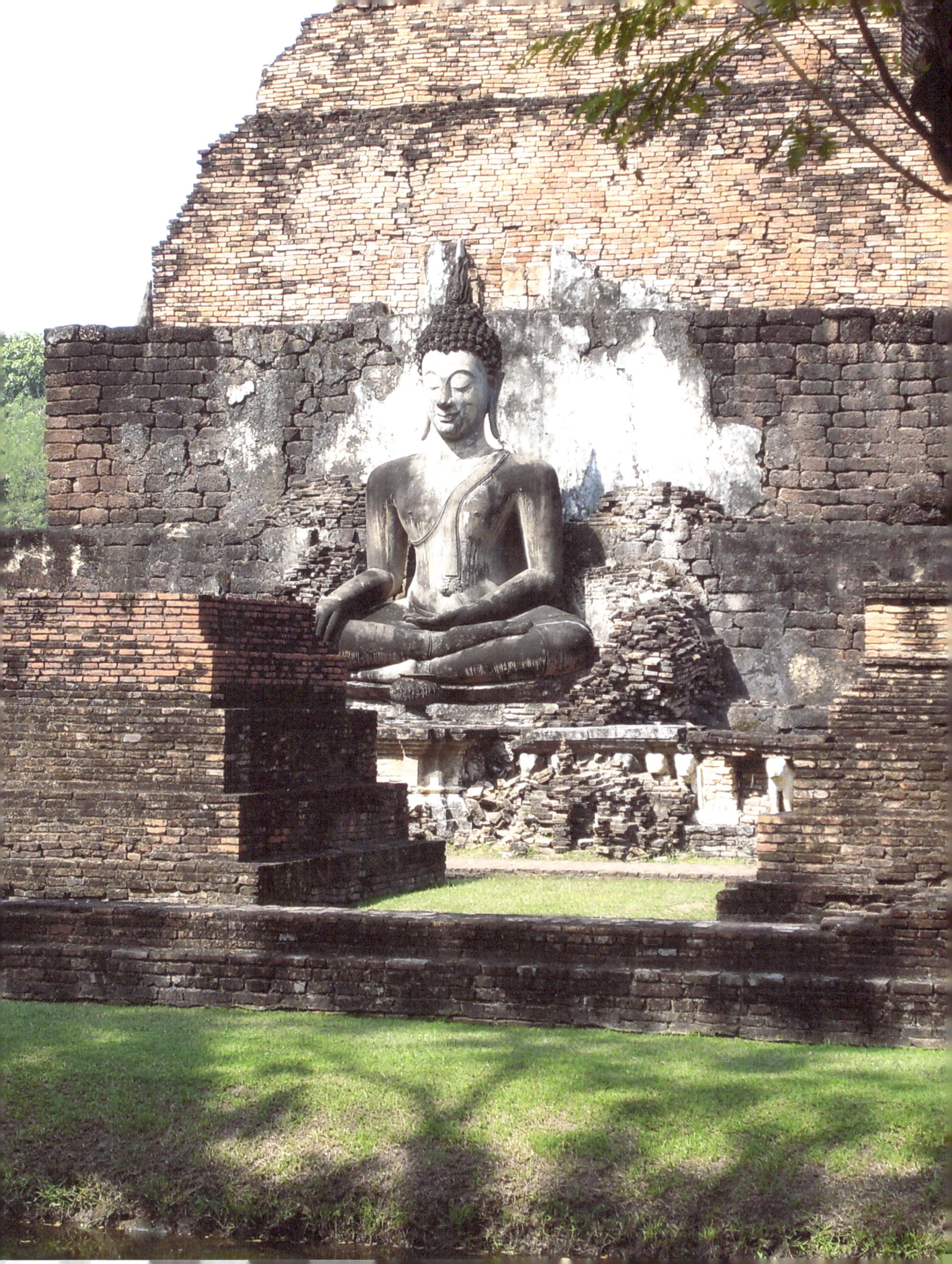

Extras

This section will address several extras that are familiar to the average Thai diet. The specific recipes I have decided to include in this first book are catered towards the western diet.

Not only should many of you should find these recipes easy to prepare but also very appetizing!

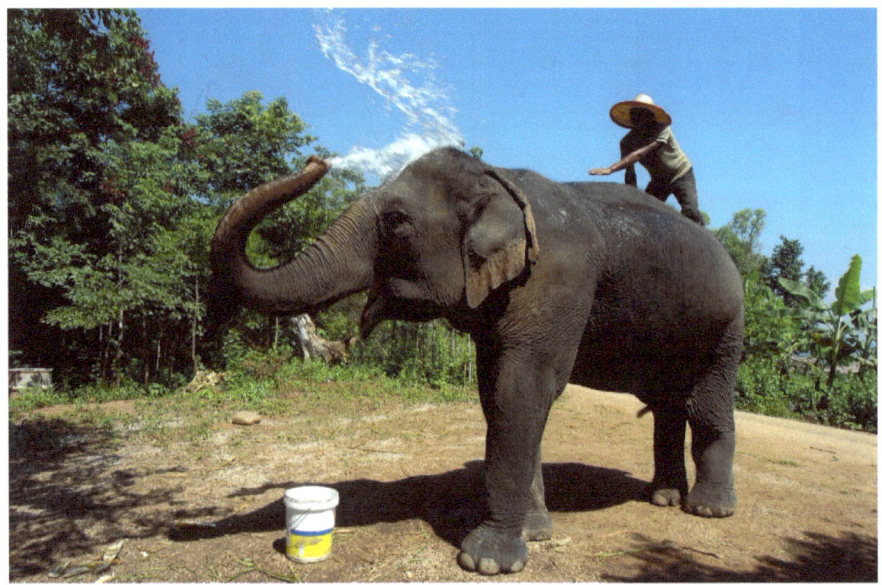

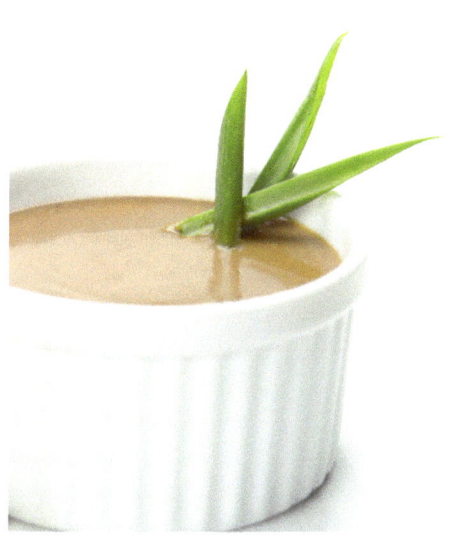

PEANUT SAUCE – is used as a dipping sauce in many Thai dishes. This recipe uses real peanuts as expected in traditional Thai dishes.

Many Non-Thai versions of this recipe will use peanut butter which dramatically changes the taste.

This recipe will serve 3 – 4 easily

Prep Time: 15 Min

Cook Time: 00 Min

2	Cups	–	Peanuts, Roasted
1/2	Cup	–	Water
2	Cloves	–	Garlic, Diced
1	Teaspoon	–	Soy Sauce
2	Teaspoons	–	Sesame Oil
3	Tablespoons	–	Light Brown Sugar
3	Tablespoons	–	Tiparos Thai Fish Sauce
1	Teaspoon	–	Tamarid Paste
1	Teaspoon	–	Chili Paste
1	Tablespoon	–	Lime Juice

Place all of the above ingredients into a blender and blend. Stop once you have reached the desired consistency.

Give the sauce a taste for preference. If it is too salty add more lime juice, and if its not salty enough add more fish sauce. Likewise add more or less chili past depending on spiciness.

Keep in mind that if the sauce is too thick it will not dip well. Add a bit more water to achieve the right consistency.

Visit www.mythaichef.com/video.html for additional tips!

THAI TEA – is very popular in Thailand and can be found on almost every street corner. This easy to make drink is great for those hot summer days.

<u>This recipe will serve 1 easily</u>   **Prep Time:** 02 Min

Cook Time: 00 Min

2	Tablespoons	–	Thai Tea
1	Tablespoon	–	Sweet Condensed Milk
1	Tablespoon	–	Sugar
1	Teaspoons	–	Milk
1	Cup	–	Hot Water

Begin by adding the sugar and condensed milk to a glass.

Put two tablespoons of Thai Tea in to a tea holder and soak the tea in the cup of hot water. Remove the tea and tea holder from the hot water and hold above the glass of sugar and condensed milk.

Continue by pouring the hot tea over the tea holder one more time into the glass.

Mix together until the sugar is completely dissolved. Add ice to cool down and pour the milk over top.

For a unique twist serve this recipe hot instead of over ice.

Visit www.mythaichef.com/video.html for additional tips!

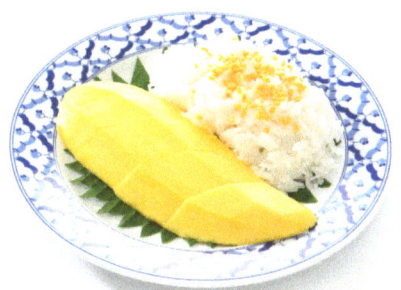

SWEET MANGO STICKY RICE – is referred to as "Khao Niaow Ma Muang" in Thai and is a great refreshing dessert.

You are sure to love this simple tropical dish.

<u>This recipe will serve 2 – 3 easily</u>

Prep Time: 10 Min

Cook Time: 25 Min

1	Cup	–	Thai Sweet Rice, Sticky Rice
1 3/4	Cup	–	Water
1	Medium	–	Mango, Cut into Pieces
1/4	Cup	–	Brown Sugar
12.5	Ounce	–	Coconut Milk
1/4	Teaspoon	–	Salt
2	Teaspoons	–	Coconut Flavoring
1	Teaspoon	–	Vanilla
2	Teaspoons	–	Cornstarch

Soak the sweet rice in 1 cup water for 30 minutes in a sauce pan. After 30 minutes stir into the rice the remaining 3/4 cup water, 1/4 can coconut milk, 1/4 tsp. salt, 1 tsp. coconut flavoring, and 1 Tbsp. brown sugar.

Place the mixture over medium high heat and bring to a slight boil. Once boiling, turn the heat to medium low and simmer.

Cook for another 10-20 minutes, or until the water has been absorbed by the rice. Remove the pot from the heat, place the lid on tight, and leave to "steam" cook for 5-10 minutes.

Prepare the sauce by adding the remaining coconut milk together with 1/4 cup sugar, 1 tsp. coconut flavoring and 1 tsp. vanilla flavoring over medium heat. This should cook for about 5 minutes.

Dissolve the cornstarch in about 2 tablespoons of water and add to the sauce stirring to thicken it slightly. As it thickens, turn down heat to low. When thickened, remove from heat.

Place scoops of the sticky rice in bowls pouring a generous amount of warm coconut sauce over the rice. Add the mango and serve.

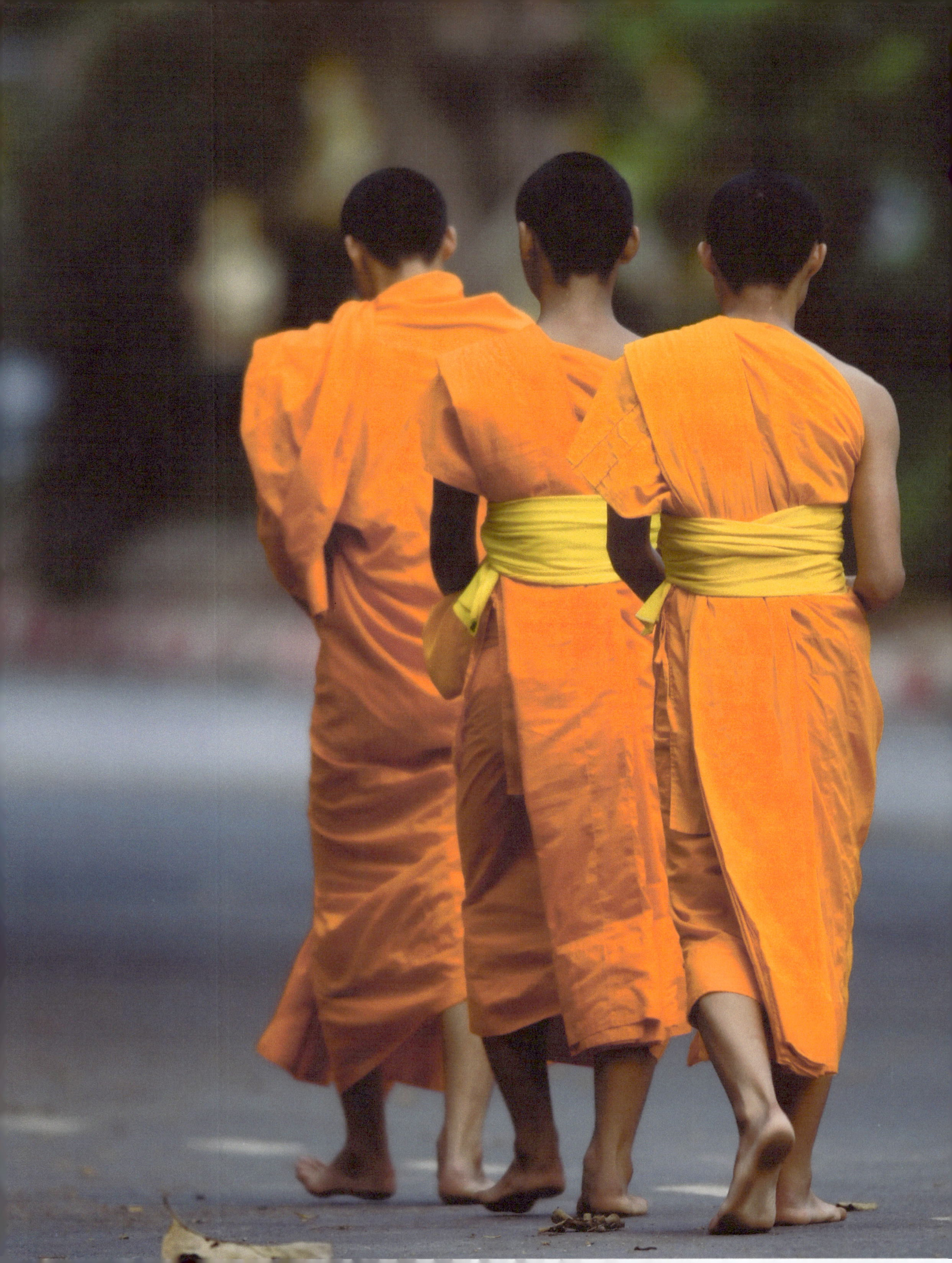

Index

A

Appetizers, 3

B

BEEF NOODLE SOUP, 26

BEEF SALAD, 18

BEEF STIR FRY, 47

C

CHICKEN FRIED RICE, 40

CHICKEN PAD THAI, 43

COCONUT CHICKEN SOUP, 22

E

Extras, 50

F

FRIED TOFU, 5

I

Introduction, 1

M

MATSAMAN CURRY, 35

Meals, 30

N

NOODLE SALAD, 16

P

PAN FRIED NOODLES, 45

PAPAYA SALAD, 12

PEANUT SAUCE, 51

PINEAPPLE FRIED RICE, 41

PINEAPPLE SHRIMP CURRY, 39

PRAWN SALAD, 14

S

Salads, 11

SATAY, 9

SCALLOPS, 6

SEAFOOD CURRY, 33

Soups, 21

SPICY CHICKEN SOUP, 23

SPICY OYSETERS, 8

SPICY SHRIMP SOUP, 25

SWEET AND SOUR CHICKEN, 48

SWEET MANGO STICKY RICE, 53

T

THAI SPICY FISH, 31

THAI SUMMER ROLLS, 4

THAI TEA, 52

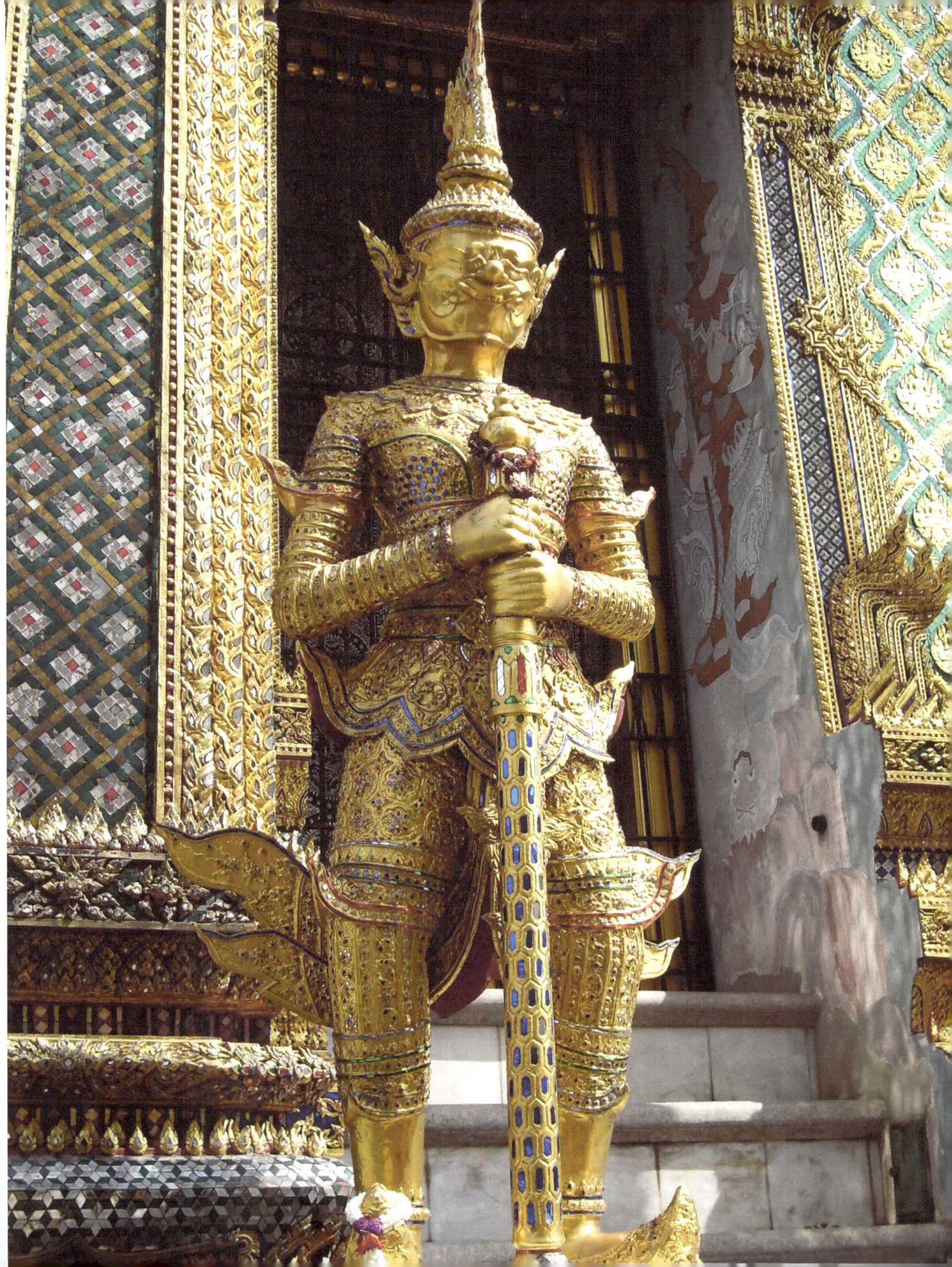

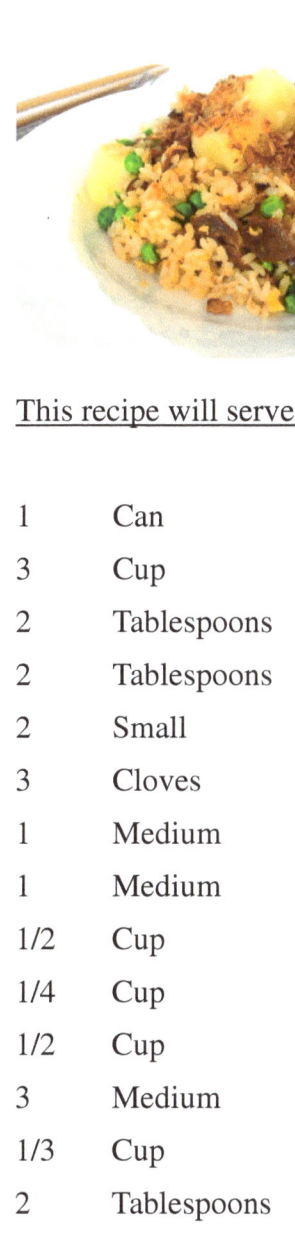

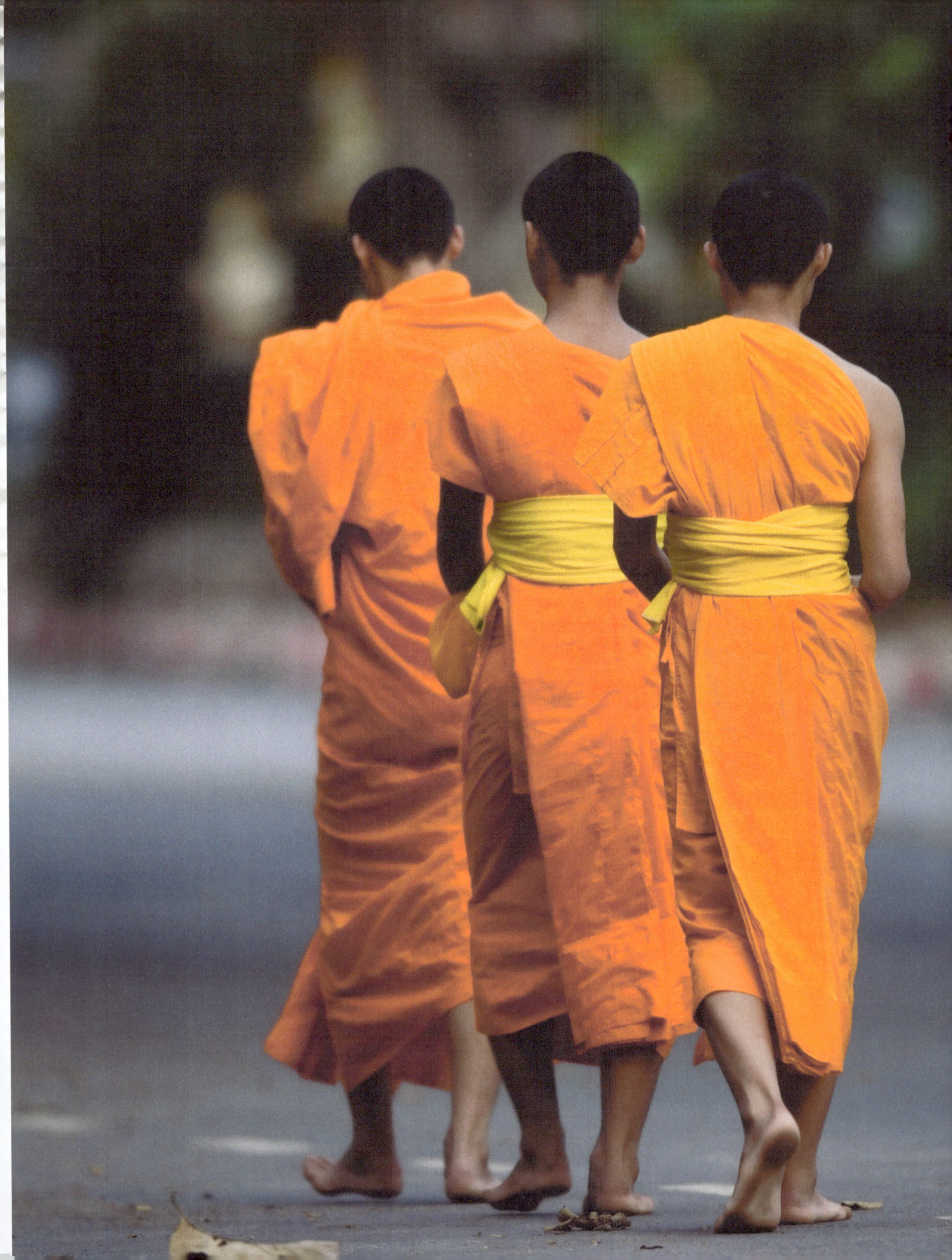

Index

A

Appetizers, 3

B

Beef Noodle Soup, 26

Beef Salad, 18

Beef Stir Fry, 47

C

Chicken Fried Rice, 40

Chicken Pad Thai, 43

Coconut Chicken Soup, 22

E

Extras, 50

F

Fried Tofu, 5

I

Introduction, 1

M

Matsaman Curry, 35

Meals, 30

N

Noodle Salad, 16

P

Pan Fried Noodles, 45

Papaya Salad, 12

Peanut Sauce, 51

Pineapple Fried Rice, 41

Pineapple Shrimp Curry, 39

Prawn Salad, 14

S

Salads, 11

Satay, 9

Scallops, 6

Seafood Curry, 33

Soups, 21

Spicy Chicken Soup, 23

Spicy Oyseters, 8

Spicy Shrimp Soup, 25

Sweet and Sour Chicken, 48

Sweet Mango Sticky Rice, 53

T

Thai Spicy Fish, 31

Thai Summer Rolls, 4

Thai Tea, 52

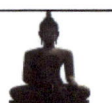
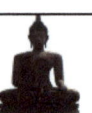

www.ingramcontent.com/pod-product-compliance
Lightning Source LLC
Chambersburg PA
CBHW041549220426
43666CB00002B/21